Drugs and Clients

What Every Psychotherapist
Needs to Know

Second Edition

Padma Catell, PhD

Solarium Press

An Imprint of Castalia Communications

Petaluma, California

Published in the United States by Solarium Press,
an imprint of Castalia Communications, Petaluma, California

www.drugsandclients.com

Library of Congress Cataloging-in-Publication Data

Catell, Padma, 1944–
  Drugs and clients: what every psychotherapist needs to know / Padma Catell.-- 1st ed.
    p. cm.
  Includes bibliographical references and index.
        ISBN 0-929150-76-7 (trade pbk.) — ISBN 0-929150-75-9 (hardcover)
  1. Psychopharmacology. 2. Mental illness--Chemotherapy.
  3. Mentally ill—Substance abuse. I. Title.
RC483.C38 2004
615'.78–dc22   2004004743

2nd Edition: Published 2010   ISBN 978-0929150-789 (trade pbk.)

_____

Credits and Permissions:

Illustrations:

Kelli Bullock: Cover, pp. 22, 54, 95, 184
Padma Catell: pp. 80, 109, 143, 199, 205, 210, 216, 220. 222, 227
Edvard Munch: "The Scream" (1893) p. 123
Sir John Tenniel, from *Alice in Wonderland* (1865) p. 159
Unknown artists: pp. 1, 41

Editing and design: Scott Morrison
Computer graphics: Jack Nau, Jerry Moffit
Copyediting: Vicki Mead

Song lyric:
"Java Jive," by Ben Oakland & Milton Drake
© 1940 (Renewed) WB Music Corp. and Sony Tunes, Inc.
All Rights Reserved   Used by Permission
WARNER BROS. PUBLICATIONS U.S. INC. Miami, FL. 33014

Zoloft® is a Registered Trademark of the Pfizer Corporation.

Manufactured in the United States of America

This book is dedicated to the memory
of my two greatest teachers,
my mother, Belle Diamond,
and Sri Brahamananda Saraswati,
who told me I would write this book
years before I ever dreamed of it.

Acknowledgements

Over the years it has taken me to write this book there have been many people who have given me help and support. It is important for me to acknowledge some to whom I am particularly grateful.

I would like to start with Ralph Metzner, dear friend and fellow traveler, since he was the one who convinced me that I could teach psychopharmacology, and it was through the process of teaching that this volume was born.

I greatly appreciate the constant love I have received from my close friends, in particular Rob Hopcke, and Wendie Brothers. Without them life would not be as funny and hard times would be much harder.

I would like to thank the "tappers," who have brought joy to my heart through dance, regardless of the pain in the other parts of my life.

I am grateful for my brother Bob, who has been, and continues to be an unfailing source of support. His love and generosity are appreciated by many, but I am the only one who has the good fortune to be able to claim him as my brother.

And finally, I want to thank my husband Scott, whose love, humor, and constancy have given me more than he can know, and without whom this book would truly never have been possible.

Table of Contents

Tables & Figures

Author's Preface

In the six years since I wrote the first edition of this book, there have been many advances in the understanding of how the brain functions and the chemistry of the central nervous system (CNS) neurons. These advances are primarily due to refinements in MRI and PET scanning techniques and the detailed information these scans provide. At the same time, few new psychoactive drugs have been introduced to the market, and a few discussed in the last edition have been removed do to safety concerns. Mainly what has happened is that, in the U.S., the Food and Drug Administration has approved new uses for drugs that were already on the market and for use in different populations than those for which the drug was originally approved. An example of this trend is the antipsychotic medication, olanzapine/Zyprexa, which is now approved for use in teenagers.

Another development has been the introduction of different variations of previously-approved drugs, such as sustained-release compounds and drugs which use a different route of administration. The primary reason for this is economic. It is much less expensive to get approval for a new use or a different formulation of a drug than it is to start from scratch and go through the many expensive levels of testing required to bring a drug to market.

The current consensus among researchers is that the drugs developed based on the knowledge of how norepinephrine (NE), serotonin (5-HT), dopamine (DA) and gamma-aminobutyric acid (GABA) affect our emotions is just about exhausted. Research is now focusing on the glutamate system and the auto receptors for the monoamines (NE, 5-HT, and DA). Even though scientists are always learning more about the CNS and its workings, the research is not yet at the point where there is enough new information for new drugs to have reached the market. Only a few drugs are now available with mechanisms of action related to these systems (e.g., memantine for Alzheimer's).

This edition includes many drugs that are still in Phase II or Phase III clinical testing that are not yet FDA approved, some of which will probably reach the market in the next few years. Drugs under study which are found to not be effective, or are found to have seriously harmful adverse effects, may never be marketed. There is no way to know which of the many drugs currently under study will be proven to be both safe and effective, receive FDA approval, and eventually reach the market.

Padma Catell, Ph.D.
April, 2010

IMPORTANT NOTICE

This book is not to be used as a guide to prescribing, taking, or discontinuing any medication, vitamin, herbal preparation, aromatherapy product, food supplement or any other substance discussed, or not discussed, herein.

Any decision as to whether to prescribe, use, or administer anything discussed or not discussed in this book must first be evaluated by a licensed, and appropriately trained, medical practitioner.

No liability will be incurred by the author or the publisher for any errors or omissions, or for any actions, either taken or not taken, by anyone regarding the material included, or not included, in this volume.

Chapter 1

Sleep & Treatment of Sleep Disorders

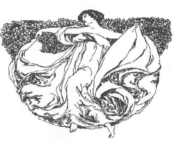

The complex process of sleep is a universal human phenomenon that both affects and reflects our psychological and physical states in profound ways. Even though its specific functions and purpose are not yet completely understood, an evaluation of a client's sleep problems and sleep patterns needs to be included as a routine part of a comprehensive psychological assessment.

Current evidence suggests that sleep is important in the consolidation of newly-learned information (Greer, 2004; Medina, 2004), in the regulation of many hormones (including thyroid hormone, leptin, and ghrelin), and that sleep deprivation may lead to weight gain (Van Cauter, et al., 2005).

It has long been known that changes in sleep patterns can be used as indicators for diagnosing anxiety and depression (Lamb, 2000; Perlis, et al., 1997). Some researchers believe that sleep disturbances may even cause these psychological disorders (Dement & Vaughan, 1999). Many psychoactive drugs cause changes in "sleep architecture" (the stages of sleep and the length of time spent in each stage) (see Fig. 1.1) (Armitage, et al., 1997; Dement & Vaughan, 1999). In the last few years, there have been significant advances in understanding that sleep disturbances indicate fundamental alterations in the functions of the *central nervous system* (CNS).

A 2008 poll released by the National Sleep Foundation reported that 65% of Americans either have trouble falling asleep, wake during the night, or wake feeling unrefreshed at least a few times each week. On average, individuals need at least eight hours of sleep. A recent finding indicates that genetic makeup may play a role in how much sleep each person needs (Gottlieb, et al., 2007).

Ten to 15% of people suffer continually from insomnia (National Sleep Foundation, 2008). The insomnia frequently lasts for days and can sometimes last for weeks. Stress, depression, anxiety, and many drugs dramatically affect our ability to sleep. Sleep problems have a very serious impact on society. The National Highway Traffic Safety Administration estimates that over 100,000 accidents every year are caused by drowsy drivers (National Sleep Foundation, 2004).

Although the specific role of sleep in health maintenance is still not clear, there is no doubt that lack of sleep can be detrimental to one's health. One large study (Dew, et al., 2003) showed that people who slept fewer than five hours per night had a 30% higher rate of heart disease than those who slept more than five hours. The research demonstrated that older adults who had periods of wakefulness of 30 minutes or more during the night had decreased longevity compared with their better-rested peers. Seniors who suffered from sleeplessness, or extremely high or low amounts of REM sleep, were about twice as likely to have died by the follow-up date (13 years later). Researchers are continuing to examine how treating older adults for sleep problems affects longevity.

A connection between sleep and depression can be seen when patients are intentionally deprived of *rapid-eye-movement* (REM) sleep (the stage when most dreaming takes place). Depressive symptoms are alleviated by one night of sleep deprivation and recur after sleeping (Seifritz, 2001). The vast majority of antidepressant medications suppress REM sleep; evidence suggests that the effectiveness for most antidepressants may be somehow connected to the suppression of REM sleep (Armitage, et al., 1997; Vogel, et al., 1990).

Bedtime and depression in teens

Researchers found that, by mandating early bedtimes for teenagers, parents may help reduce their teens' risk for depression and suicidal thoughts. A study of 15,000 teenagers found that those with bedtimes of midnight or later were 25% more likely to suffer from depression and 20% more likely to have suicidal thoughts than their better-rested peers. This study supports the idea that inadequate sleep may lead to depression (Gangwisch, 2009).

Though the details of the relationship between mental disorders and sleep are not yet understood, it is clear that a strong connection exists. A better understanding of this relationship could lead to new treatments for both psychological problems and sleep disorders.

Normal Sleep & the Sleep Cycle

To understand sleep disorders, it is important to understand the patterns of the normal sleep cycle (see Fig. 1.1) (Dement & Vaughn, 1999; Doghramji, 1989; Loomis, et al., 1937; National Sleep Foundation, 2004; Roehrs, 2000; Roth, et al., 1994). It takes an average of 30 to 45 minutes after falling asleep to progress from Stage 1 to Delta sleep.

One then passes back from Delta to Stage 1. At this point the first period of REM sleep usually occurs. For most people, REM begins approximately 90 minutes after falling asleep (Dement & Vaughan, 1999). The period between falling asleep and the first onset of REM is termed *REM latency* (Doghramji, 1989; Hauri & Orr, 1982). The duration of REM latency can be useful as a diagnostic measure for depressive, sleep, and anxiety disorders.

The percentage of time spent in REM sleep declines with age. REM takes up about 80% of life for an infant who is born prematurely and about 50% for a full-term newborn. Young and middle-aged adults spend 20% of their sleep in REM, and the elderly only 15% (Hauri & Orr, 1982; Perlis, et al., 1997).

Most dreaming takes place during REM sleep, and some dreaming occurs during Delta sleep. We usually do not remember dreams that take place during Delta. When awakened from REM, people can recall dreams about 80% of the time. As sleep progresses through the night, the periods of REM sleep become more frequent, each episode of REM lasts longer, and the time between REM episodes decreases.

The electroencephalogram (EEG) readings becomes increasingly slower and more synchronized as one progresses from Stage 1 to Delta sleep. During Delta the *parasympathetic nervous system* (PSNS), which controls homeostatic functions, dominates. There is an increase in gastrointestinal (GI) motility (movement), large muscles relax (although there are some small body movements), heart rate slows, blood pressure decreases, and respiration rate slows and becomes more even (Kandel & Schwartz, 1981).

The phenomena of both sleepwalking and *night terrors* (when children scream in their sleep and seem to be having terrifying dreams from which it is difficult to awaken them) occur during Delta sleep. The length of time spent in each period of Delta becomes shorter as the night progresses. For most people, sleep becomes "lighter" toward the morning, and awakenings are more frequent (Kandel & Schwartz, 1981). Although this sleep pattern is the norm, there are many individual differences. Some people report that they sleep more deeply toward morning.

Delta sleep may disappear completely in people over age 60 (Dement & Vaughan, 1999). This progressive decrease in Delta sleep contributes to the increase in insomnia and the many spontaneous awakenings experienced by the elderly.

Stages of Sleep

The stages of sleep were first described in 1937 as defined by changes in EEG patterns (Loomis, et al., 1937). Body movements and eye movements may also be specific to the various sleep stages.

Sleep latency

This is the period between lying down and closing one's eyes and the start of Stage 1 sleep (on average about 10 to 15 minutes) (Hauri & Orr, 1982).

Stage 1

The initial stage of sleep is relatively brief, usually between 30 seconds and 7 minutes. Reactivity to outside stimuli is diminished, thoughts begin to drift, and short dreams may take place. The EEG will indicate brain waves in the theta range, which is between three and seven cycles per second (cps) (Hauri & Orr, 1982).

Stage 2

During this stage mental processes consist of short, fragmented thoughts. Stage 2 is marked by the appearance on the EEG of a pattern known as "sleep spindles." These spindles denote bursts of brain activity in the 12 to 14 cps range, each lasting between one-half second and two seconds. This stage occurs repeatedly throughout the night (Hauri & Orr, 1982).

Delta

Delta is the "deepest" stage of sleep and combines what was historically known as Stage 3 and Stage 4 sleep. This stage is distinguished by the presence of delta waves on the EEG. Delta waves are one-half to two cps and have high amplitudes. This slow-frequency, high-amplitude pattern must exist in at least 20% of the EEG for the stage to be designated as Delta sleep. Because of these slow waves seen on the EEG this is also called "slow wave" or "deep sleep." It is difficult to be awakened from Delta sleep. The percentage of time spent in Delta decreases with age. Research has shown that by the time men reach the age of 45 many have nearly lost their ability to fall into deep (Delta) sleep (Hauri & Orr, 1982).

Normal Sleep Architecture

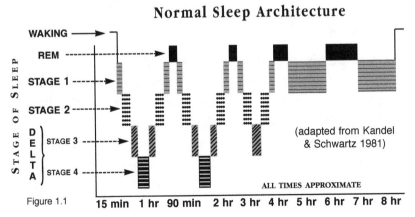

Figure 1.1

Rapid-eye movement (REM) sleep

REM sleep resembles Stage 1 in its EEG pattern. During REM, the EEG becomes desynchronized and shows waves of higher frequency and lower voltage than in the other stages of sleep. EEG patterns are similar to the wakeful state. REM sleep can be further separated into *tonic* and *phasic* components which are physiologically distinct from each other. Tonic REM is characterized by muscle paralysis in skeletal muscles, increased cerebral blood flow, and an increase in brain temperature. Phasic REM includes short episodes of rapid-eye movement and muscle twitching; the body appears highly activated. REM sleep is when most dreaming takes place. Its closeness to the waking state facilitates one's ability to remember dreams. Contrary to popular belief, REM is not a "deep" stage of sleep (Delta). One can easily be awakened during REM sleep (Hauri & Orr, 1982).

Effects of Drugs on Sleep Architecture

Benzodiazepines/benzodiazepine receptor agonists (BzRAs)

Delta sleep is reduced by benzodiazepines (e.g., diazepam/Valium, alprazolam/Xanax) much more than is REM sleep. This reduction in Delta leads to a decrease in night terrors and some nightmares. BzRAs are used to treat these disorders since they decrease and eventually eliminate the stage of sleep when these disturbances occur (Armitage, et al., 1997). (For a definition of *agonist* see Appendix E.)

Selective serotonin reuptake inhibitors (SSRIs)

Research shows that because it reduces deep (Delta) sleep, the antidepressant paroxetine/Paxil (and probably all the SSRIs) can be helpful in treatment of night terrors (Armitage, et al., 1997).

Also, if someone is not sleeping due to anxiety, taking an SSRI may reduce the anxiety which may lead to an easier time falling asleep and staying asleep.

Alcohol & barbiturates

Chronic use of both alcohol and barbiturates causes a suppression of REM sleep. Barbiturate use leads to an increase in Stage 2 sleep and a decrease in Delta sleep (Kandel & Schwartz, 1981). People with a history of drug or alcohol abuse may report sleep disturbances for many years after cessation of the drug or alcohol use. Chronic alcohol use seems to impair processes that allow restorative sleep to make up for sleep deprivation. This may be due to interference with a sleep dependent rhythm (known as "process S") that increases the amount of slow-wave sleep (Irwin, et al., 2002). Problems with falling asleep and a decrease in slow-wave sleep are seen frequently during abstinence after habitual alcohol use. An antiseizure drug, gabapentin/Neurontin, has been found to be the best treatment for this type of insomnia (Karam-Hage, 2004).

REM rebound

REM rebound is the increase in time spent in REM sleep following a period of REM deprivation. Most likely it is the body's attempt to maintain homeostasis. Its duration varies from person to person, and is related to the extent of the REM deprivation. REM rebound is marked by an increase in the number of spontaneous awakenings during the night and by an increase in restlessness and dreaming. A person may feel sleep deprived during REM rebound due to the corresponding decrease in Delta sleep. No serious mental problems seem to be caused by REM sleep deprivation.

Neurotransmitters & Neuromodulators in Sleep

Wakefulness and sleep are discrete processes mediated by different substances in the central nervous system (Roehrs, 2000; Stahl, 1999). Many drugs, by affecting specific *neurotransmitters* (NTs) and *neuromodulators* (NMs), cause changes in sleep patterns. These NTs and NMs, in addition to their involvement in sleep and wakefulness, have a role in many processes in the CNS, including various mental and emotional states.

Serotonin (5-HT, 5-hydroxytryptamine)

Serotonin (5-HT) seems to be the neuromodulator most involved in sleep induction. Taking 5-HT precursors (the amino acid tryptophan or 5-HTP {5-hydroxytryptophan}) leads to an increase in 5-HT synthesis, which facilitates the ability to fall asleep.

Norepinephrine (NE)

The presence of norepinephrine (NE) seems to be related to alertness and symptoms of anxiety. NE is known to have a role in the symptoms of depression, which also affects sleep patterns.

Dopamine (DA)

Dopamine (DA) is involved in reward processes, pleasurable states, and normal movement. DA seems to stimulate reward centers in the CNS. Stimulation of DA receptors is increased when stimulant drugs like cocaine or methamphetamine are taken.

Hypocretin-1 & hypocretin-2 (orexins)

These chemicals are found in the *hypothalamus*, the part of the brain that regulates sleep and the endocrine system. It is postulated that hypocretin is necessary to maintain a non-REM state. Levels of hypocretin are low in humans with narcolepsy and are completely absent in the narcoleptic dogs used in studies of sleep disorders (Lin, et al., 1999).

Acetylcholine (ACh)

The neurotransmitter acetylcholine (ACh) has a role in REM and Delta sleep. Experiments show that the firing of acetylcholine neurons increases during Delta sleep and increases even more during REM sleep (Dement & Vaughan, 1999).

Melatonin

Melatonin is involved in the process of falling asleep. Its secretion is responsive to cycles of light and darkness. Its release is inhibited by light and increased by darkness (Dement & Vaughan, 1999).

Sleep Disorders

Disorders of initiating & maintaining sleep

Sleep problems are frequently seen in conjunction with affective (mood), personality, and somatoform (involving the body) disorders. Treatment for these may include analytic psychotherapy and behavioral therapy, either alone or in combination with various psychoactive compounds such as sedative, *anxiolytic* (anxiety decreasing), antidepressant, and antimanic medications (see Chapters 2, 4, and 5 for detailed discussions of these compounds).

Non-prescription treatments for insomnia

Many alternative treatments for insomnia are currently being tried. Some nutritional supplements are known to aid sleep:

- Calcium: For adults, 600 mg taken at bedtime
- Magnesium: 250 mg taken at bedtime
- Vitamin B_6: 50 to 100 mg/day may prevent insomnia
- Vitamin B_{12}: 25 mg supplemented with 100 mg of vitamin B_5 can serve as an effective anti-insomnia regimen (Alternative sleep aids, 2004).

(See Chapter 11 for more information on aromatherapy and herbal treatments for insomnia.)

Disorders of excessive somnolence

People who suffer from these disorders have the experience of getting lots of sleep, yet they always feel sleepy (Hauri & Orr, 1982).

NARCOLEPSY

Narcolepsy is due to abnormal occurrences of REM sleep. Symptoms of narcolepsy, such as taking frequent naps and excessive sleepiness, can easily be misdiagnosed as a lack of motivation or as depression. Between 50,000 and 250,000 people in the United States suffer from narcolepsy. Narcolepsy occurs about as frequently as *multiple sclerosis* (MS). Males and females are affected equally, and there is strong evidence that narcolepsy has a genetic component. The relatives of narcoleptics are much more likely to develop this disorder than the average person (Dement & Vaughan, 1999).

Although this is changing, most sleep researchers believe that narcolepsy is still greatly underdiagnosed (National Sleep Foundation, 2004). A definitive diagnosis usually requires spending one to three nights in a sleep laboratory for brain-wave (EEG) pattern monitoring during sleep (Dement & Vaughan, 1999). These diagnostic procedures are expensive and sleep laboratories are still scarce; both factors contribute to the under-diagnosis of narcolepsy.

A person who suffers from narcolepsy goes directly into REM sleep rather than progressing through the other stages of sleep before going into the first REM period (Doghramji, 1989) (see Fig. 1.1). Going directly into REM causes the symptoms of *cataplexy*, sleep paralysis, and hypnogogic hallucinations (see below).

Recognizing the symptoms of narcolepsy is important for the psychotherapist because these symptoms can easily be confused with depression and because psychoactive medication is usually a component of the treatment. When narcolepsy is suspected, referral to a psychiatrist for a diagnosis and a medication evaluation is always necessary.

Etiology of narcolepsy

Narcolepsy is believed to be an inherited neurological disorder that manifests as an abnormally high incidence of REM sleep. Researchers have discovered a specific neurotransmitter, hypocretin, which seems to be necessary to keep one awake (Hungs & Mignot, 2001). Hypocretin is produced primarily by cells in the hypothalamus. These cells are missing or damaged in people with narcolepsy. There is some evidence that the damage may be due to an autoimmune reaction (Hungs & Mignot, 2001; Lin, et al., 1999; Scammell, et al., 2000).

Symptoms of narcolepsy

On occasion, everyone experiences some of the symptoms of

narcolepsy. A diagnosis of narcolepsy requires at least four of the symptoms described below or the presence of cataplexy. Even when many symptoms are present, analysis by a sleep expert is essential for a definitive diagnosis.

Symptoms usually begin between the ages of 10 and 20. They generally reach a plateau in severity and then remain constant. The disorder typically lasts for life. Many patients report that they gain better control over their symptoms as they get older (National Sleep Foundation, 2004). Usually, the first two symptoms experienced are *sleep attacks* and *excessive daytime sleepiness* (EDS). Cataplexy may develop early in the disease, simultaneously with sleep attacks and daytime sleepiness, although in some people cataplexy does not appear until many years after the initial symptoms (Dement & Vaughan, 1999).

Excessive daytime sleepiness (EDS)

Excessive daytime sleepiness affects approximately 250,000 Americans every year. EDS can be experienced either by itself or as a symptom of narcolepsy, sleep apnea, or other disorders. With narcolepsy, EDS usually develops over a period of several years. The first symptoms of EDS are usually an increase in sleepiness and sleep attacks (see below) (Dement & Vaughan, 1999). EDS indicates actual sleepiness (as differentiated from fatigue, depression, or lack of energy). An EDS sufferer has sudden episodes of sleepiness, often at highly inappropriate times, such as when driving, eating, or having sex. Episodes occur on an almost daily basis. On average, someone with EDS will only take five minutes to fall asleep (compared with ten minutes or more for most people) (Hauri & Orr, 1982).

Symptoms of EDS may indicate a serious organic disorder, usually either narcolepsy or sleep apnea. Many psychological conditions, such as depression, may have fatigue as a symptom. Until recently, an accurate diagnosis for sleep apnea required a costly night or two in a sleep lab. Due to new technology, a patient can now sleep at home while connected to a recorder and have the result evaluated by a sleep expert at a later time.

Sleep attacks

Sleep attacks are the tendency to fall asleep in situations in which many people might feel sleepy, such as after a meal, or while listening to a boring speaker. These attacks are a manifestation of going directly into REM without first passing through the other stages of sleep (Dement & Vaughan, 1999).

With narcolepsy, sleep attacks increase in frequency and begin to occur in situations that are less usual for people who are not affected by this disorder, such as while reading a newspaper, writing a letter, or waiting in line at a store. After a while, a person who has narcolepsy begins to fall asleep at times that are even less appropriate, such as while driving a car or in the middle of a conversation.

Each sleep attack can last from a few seconds to about 15 minutes. Often, the person may not realize he or she has been asleep and may behave oddly upon awakening, such as continuing a conversation or activity exactly where they left off (Dement & Vaughan, 1999). During a sleep attack, a dream may be perceived as a real event because the person has no internal awareness of the period of sleep. The experience can be very confusing, both for the person with narcolepsy and for anyone who happens to be nearby.

Pramipexole/Mirapex and ropinirole/Requip, two drugs used to treat Parkinson's disease, have been found to cause sleep attacks (Kandel & Schwartz, 1981). Sleep attacks brought on by these drugs have occurred while patients were driving and have resulted in accidents. Because it is impossible to predict which patients on these drugs are most likely to experience sleep attacks, it is recommended that people using these medications do not drive. The attacks cease when the drugs are discontinued.

Cataplexy

Cataplexy is a short episode, usually lasting a few seconds to 30 minutes, in which there is a decrease or a complete loss of voluntary muscle control. This symptom is caused by going directly into a period of REM and experiencing the corresponding muscle paralysis (tonic REM). Severity can range from slight feelings of muscle weakness to a state of collapse involving all voluntary muscles.

Cataplectic attacks can be brought on by emotion, stress, or fatigue. (Examples of cataplexy can be viewed on YouTube.) The most frequent cause is when experiencing strong emotion, in particular laughter and anger, but an attack can be triggered by a stimulus as minor as the memory of an emotional situation. At first, cataplectic attacks are usually mild and infrequent; generally, they will progress in severity and frequency until they reach a plateau. The intensity of the episodes may vary from one attack to the next. The frequency of the attacks differs from person to person; they may range from one or two per year to hundreds of attacks each day. A cataplectic attack may develop into a sleep attack if the person is reclining or sitting. The sufferer remains aware of his or her surroundings; this differentiates cataplexy from a seizure. The presence of cataplexy in narcolepsy ranges from 65% to 90%. Cataplexy is a definitive indicator for a diagnosis of narcolepsy (Dement & Vaughan, 1999).

Automatic behavior

Automatic behavior is when a person does something and subsequently has no conscious recollection of having done it (e.g., driving somewhere and having no memory of how one got there, or putting dirty dishes in the clothes dryer and being awakened by the sound of the breaking dishes). To a casual observer, automatic behavior may not seem noteworthy or appear any different from normal activity. People suffering from it may be aware of a blank space in their memory during these periods. This symptom can be a source of confusion or shame, particularly if it is not recognized as caused by narcolepsy (Dement & Vaughan, 1999).

Sleep paralysis

Sleep paralysis is an inability to move that usually occurs either during the transition between sleep and waking, when falling asleep, or while waking up. Common feelings are being unable to open one's eyes, speak, or move. The experience is generally frightening. It is often described as feeling paralyzed coupled with the fear that there is a menacing figure nearby intent on doing one harm. There is usually complete recall of the episode after waking. Sleep paralysis is a common experience for many people who do not have narcolepsy or any other disorder.

Hypnogogic hallucinations

Hypnogogic hallucinations are vivid, brief dreams that occur when falling asleep. The hallucinations are so brief that there may be difficulty distinguishing them from the waking state.

Sleep apnea with narcolepsy

People with narcolepsy often have other sleep disorders. About 20% of male narcoleptic patients also have sleep apnea (see below) (National Sleep Foundation, 2004).

Treatment of narcolepsy

Although there is currently no cure for narcolepsy, the symptoms can be somewhat controlled with psychoactive medications. Gamma-hydroxybutyric acid (GHB)/Xyrem is a sedative drug that is believed to help with the symptoms of narcolepsy (particularly cataplexy) by regulating sleep architecture (Robinson & Keating, 2007). Since many of the symptoms of narcolepsy are made worse by irregular sleep cycles at night, regulation of sleep during the night will decrease symptoms of sleepiness during the day. Because GHB has been abused (the "date rape" drug) it is currently being dispensed by only one pharmacy in the U.S. and physicians must determine that their patients meet very specific criteria before the drug is dispensed. As time passes, if there is no evidence of an increase in abuse, these restrictions will probably lessen. Xyrem comes in liquid form and its effects last for only four hours. For this reason, people with narcolepsy have to take a second dose during the night to have their sleep cycles regulated for eight hours (Borgen, et al., 2002). Xyrem is believed to consolidate sleep, reduce cataplectic attacks, and reduce the severity of EDS.

Drugs such as modafinil/Provigil (which was developed and approved specifically to treat narcolepsy) and the mixed stimulant drugs (such as amphetamines/Adderall and methylphenidate/Ritalin) decrease excessive sleepiness (Scammell, et al., 2000). All of these drugs have the potential for abuse.

Since antidepressant medications suppress REM sleep, they can be used to treat attacks of cataplexy, sleep paralysis, and hypnogogic hallucinations (Vogel, et al., 1990). Taking naps during the day and avoiding alcohol and other CNS depressants (which change sleep architecture) can also be helpful in alleviating symptoms.

REM SLEEP BEHAVIOR DISORDER

This disorder is the result of a breakdown in the brain process that prevents motor activity during REM sleep (see p. 6). This breakdown allows the movement of large muscles during dreaming. The usual symptoms are kicking, punching, arm-swinging, and other movements that seem to be the acting out of dreams.

Over 90% of those affected with REM sleep behavior disorder are men over the age of 50. There is some evidence that it is associated with narcolepsy, Parkinson's disease, Lewy body disease, and multiple-system atrophy. This disorder may be the first sign of the presence of some neurological disease (Portet & Touchon, 2002). Clonazepam (a BzRA which interferes with REM sleep) is used to decrease the symptoms of REM sleep behavior disorder.

SLEEP APNEA

Sleep apnea is a common cause of disrupted sleep and affects about 4% of men and 2% of women. The apnea is a suspension of breathing that can last from 10 to 120 seconds and is marked by heavy snoring and a struggle to breathe. It occurs when the upper airway collapses repeatedly during sleep. After a while, the person becomes semi-awake and breathing resumes. The diagnosis of apnea requires more than 75 awakenings per night (some people experience hundreds of episodes of awakening during a single night).

A sufferer may have no specific awareness of the apnea, but the next day may feel excessively sleepy, have difficulty concentrating, and have no idea as to the cause. Frequently, it is the partner of someone with apnea who notices something is wrong, becomes frightened by the irregular breathing or gasping during the night, and requests that their partner be evaluated by a physician.

Because of their sleep-deprived state, those with apnea are six times more likely to have traffic accidents. Often life-style changes, like losing weight, quitting smoking, and avoiding alcohol and/or sleeping pills will decrease the episodes. This type of apnea is usually effectively treated with a device that provides *continuous positive air pressure* (CPAP or BiPAP) or with laser surgery to open up the airway.

SLEEP HYGIENE

Stanford's Dr. Clete Kushida, president of the American Academy of Sleep Medicine, who has worked in the field of sleep research since 1977, offers these tips to a better night's sleep:

- Maintain a regular schedule. Go to bed and rise at the same time as consistently as possible each day and select the number of hours of sleep that make you feel best, whether seven hours or 10.

- Use bright light within five minutes of waking, for 30 minutes, to synchronize your internal clock.

- Avoid bright light two to three hours before bedtime (as this delays sleep onset). If you read, use just enough light and avoid halogen lights.

- Avoid remaining in bed if you can't sleep. After 20 minutes, if you can't sleep or fall back asleep, go into another room and do something else until you feel drowsy.

- Avoid reading or watching TV in bed (especially thriller novels or action shows) unless this makes you drowsy.
- Avoid napping, unless you nap every day at the same time for the same amount of time, or you are tired and about to get behind the wheel of a car.

For more information, or to read more on insomnia, go to Stanford Professor Dr. Rachel Manber's paper at knol.google.com/k/Rachel-manber/insomnia (Zinko, 2009) or consult *The Promise of Sleep,* by William Dement, MD, which is an excellent book for anyone who is interested in this topic.

Direct Relevance to Psychotherapy

Feeling rested contributes to a state of psychological and physical well-being. Psychotherapists need to inquire about their clients' sleep habits and assess for possible problems. Even in so-called "normal" aging there is an increase in sleep difficulties. People often do not realize that anxiety and depression affect sleep patterns, and often they do not report difficulties or changes in sleep to their therapists. Many clients may not mention that they are taking some form of sleep aid on a daily or as-needed basis. Clients may consume a wide range of products reputed to aid in falling asleep or staying asleep, including herbal teas, over-the-counter sleep medications, prescription sedatives or antianxiety drugs, the hormone melatonin, the amino acid trypto-phan, and others. Many people are dependent on some type of sleep aid to obtain what they think of as "a good night's sleep."

The psychotherapist needs to assess the client's level of knowledge about normal sleep patterns and whether there is an understanding of the changes that take place with age. The psychotherapist can also gather information as to whether medications are being taken that might affect the client's sleep patterns (sedatives or stimulants) and give feedback about this to both the client and to the prescribing physician. The psychotherapist may be in the best position to synthesize all the pieces of information and consult with the client and the physician to determine what can be done to help the client achieve a more restful night's sleep and a better understanding of the sleep process.

Appropriate treatment always depends upon accurate diagnosis. Psychological treatments and medications used to alleviate symptoms may differ greatly depending upon whether the underlying cause of the sleep problem is a psychosis, depression, or anxiety. Whenever possible, interventions should address underlying disorders rather than just alleviate symptoms. If the underlying cause is treated, the sleep problem is also usually alleviated. An accurate diagnosis is particularly critical if medication is to be a component of the client's treatment. Without a complete psychological assessment, treating the sleep disorder with medication or herbal products can worsen both the sleep disorder and the psychological condition.

In general, anxiety is correlated with difficulty falling asleep, whereas depression is correlated with early morning awakening. If difficulty falling asleep is due to an underlying anxiety disorder, treatment with an antianxiety medication or an SSRI might be the most appropriate pharmacological intervention (Armitage, et al., 1997). (See Chapter 2.)

About 70% of patients with insomnia have depression as the underlying cause. The remaining 30% have other sleep disorders. If the sleep problem is caused by depression, then taking BzRAs (see Table 2.1) may actually worsen the depression, and over time can increase sleep difficulties (National Sleep Foundation, 2004). Treatment with an antidepressant (usually an SSRI) is a more appropriate intervention in these cases.

Taking sleep medication every night is not recommended. Certain BzRAs classified as *hypnotics* (triazolam, flurazepam, temazepam) are helpful with sleep problems if taken for less than two weeks, or if not used more than three nights in a row. If taken longer or more frequently, sleep architecture will be adversely altered (Vogel, et al., 1990).

An acute psychotic episode is often accompanied by sleep problems. When psychotic symptoms are present, a specific diagnosis is critical before medications are chosen. The presence of hallucinations, feelings of persecution and other fears, can frequently lead to sleep disturbances.

There can also be sleep disturbances with no underlying psychological problem. For example, due to individual sleep rhythms, one person may not be able to sleep during the night, may fall asleep in the early morning, and may sleep until mid-day. These patterns can be relatively easy to modify. The most appropriate treatment may be education in techniques of basic sleep hygiene. Many good books are available on this topic (Bootzin & Perlis; 1992, Dement & Vaughan, 1999; Idzikowski, 2000).

It is very common for a client to have some type of sleep disorder along with various psychological problems. A client may be taking medication for both the sleep disorder and the psychological disorder. For optimal treatment, it is important for the psychotherapist to consult with the prescribing physician whenever a client is on psychoactive medications and a sleep disorder is a presenting problem.

References for Chapter 1

Alternative sleep aids. Retrieved April, 9, 2004, from
　　http://www.healingdeva.com/selena2.htmSuggestedSupplements
Armitage, R., Yonkers, K., Cole, D. & Rush, J. (1997). A multicenter, double-blind comparison of the effects of nefazodone and fluoxetine on sleep architecture and quality of sleep in depressed outpatients. *J. Clinical Psychopharm.*, 17(3), 161–168.
Bootzin, R. & Perlis, M. (1992). Nonpharmacological treatments of insomnia. *J. Clinical Psychiatry,* 53, 37–41.
Borgen, L., Cook, H., Hornfeldt, C. & Fuller, D. (2002). Sodium Oxybate (GHB) for treatment of cataplexy. *Pharmacotherapy,* 22(6), 798–799.
Dement, W. & Vaughan, C. (1999). *The Promise of Sleep: A Pioneer in Sleep Medicine Explores the Vital Connection Between Health, Happiness, and a Good Night's Sleep.* New York, NY: Delacorte Press.
Dew, M., Hoch, C., Buysse, D., Monk, T., Begley, A., Houck, P., Hall, M., Kupfer, D. & Reynolds, C. (2003). Healthy older adults' sleep predicts all-cause mortality at 4 to 19 years of follow up. *Psychosomatic Medicine,* 65, 63–73.

Doghramji, K. (1989). Sleep disorders: A selective update. *Hospital and Community Psychiatry*, 40(1), 29–40.

Gangwisch, J. (2009). Earlier parental mandated bedtimes for adolescents as a protective factor against depression and suicidal ideation as mediated by sleep duration. *Sleep 2009*, the 23rd Annual Meeting of the Associated Professional Sleep Societies.

Gottlieb, D., O'Connor, G. & Wilk, J. (2007). Genome-wide association of sleep and circadian phenotypes. *BMC Medical Genetics*, 8(Suppl. 1), S9.

Greer, M. (2004). Strengthen your brain by resting it. *Monitor on Psychology*, July/August, 60-62.

Hauri, P. & Orr, W. (1982). *The Sleep Disorders*. Upjohn Co., Kalamazoo, MI.

Hungs, M. & Mignot, E. (2001). Hypocretin/orexin, sleep and narcolepsy. *Bioessays*, 23, 397–408.

Idzikowski, C. (2000). *Learn to Sleep Well*. London: Duncan Baird.

Irwin, M., Gillin, J., Dang, J., Weissman, J., Phillips, E. & Ehlers, C. (2002). Sleep deprivation as a probe of homeostatic sleep regulation in primary alcoholics. *Biol. Psych.*, 51(8), 632-41.

Kandel, E. & Schwartz, J. (1981). *Principles of Neuroscience*. New York: Elsevier North Holland, Inc.

Karam-Hage, M. (2004). Treating insomnia in patients with substance use/abuse Disorders. *Psychiatric Times*, February, 55–56.

Lamb, M. (2000). Is it just insomnia? *Psychology Today*, March/April, 14.

Lin, L., Faraco, J., Li, R., Kadotani, H., Rogers, W., Lin, X., Qui, X. & de Jong, P. (1999). The sleep disorder canine narcolepsy is caused by a mutation in the hypocretin (orexin) receptor 2 gene. *Cell*, 98, 365–376.

Loomis, A., Harvey, E. & Hobart, G. (1937). Cerebral states during sleep, as studied by human brain potentials. *J. Exp. Psychol.*, 21, 127–44.

Medina, J. (2004), Why do we need to sleep? *Psychiatric Times*, September, 27-29.

National Sleep Foundation. (2004). 888-NSF-SLEEP. Retrieved from http://www.sleepfoundation.org/ Information on sleep disorders and sleep disorder clinics.

National Sleep Foundation (2008). 888-NSF-SLEEP. Retrieved from http://www.sleepfoundation.org/ Information on sleep disorders and sleep disorder clinics.

Perlis, M., Giles, D., Buysse, D., Tu, X. & Kupfer, D. (1997). Self-reported sleep disturbance as a prodromal symptom in recurrent depression. *J. Affective Disorders*, 42(2–3), 209–212.

Portet, F. & Touchon, J. (2002). REM Sleep behavioral disorder. *Rev. Neurol.* (Paris), 158(11), 1049-56.

Robinson, D. & Keating, G. (2007). Sodium oxybate: A review of its use in the management of narcolepsy. *CNS Drugs*, 21(4), 337-354.

Roehrs, T. (2000). Sleep physiology and pathophysiology. *Clinical Cornerstone*, 2(5), 1–15.

Roth, T., Roehrs, T., Carskadon, M. & Dement, W. (1994). Daytime sleepiness and alertness. In M. H. Kryger, T. Roth & W. C. Dement (Eds.). *Principals and Practice of Sleep Medicine*. Philadelphia: W. B. Saunders Co.

Scammell, T., Estabrooke, I., McCarthy, M., Chemelli, R., Yanagisawa, M., Miller, M. S., & Saper, C. (2000). Hypothalamic arousal regions are activated during modafinil-induced wakefulness. *J. Neuroscience*, 20, 8620–8.

Seifritz, E. (2001). Contribution of sleep physiology to depressive pathophysiology. *Neuropsychopharm.*, 25, 585–588.

Stahl, S. (1999). Awakening to the psychopharmacology of sleep and arousal: Novel neurotransmitters and wake-promoting drugs. *J. Clinical Psychiatry*, 63(4), 339–402.

Van Cauter, E., Knutson, K., Leproult, R. & Spiegel, K. (2005). The Impact of Sleep Deprivation on Hormones and Metabolism. *Medscape Neurology & Neurosurgery*. Insomnia and Sleep Health Expert Column, April 28. 2005. Retrieved December 26, 2009 <http://cme.medscape.com/viewarticle/502825?rss>http://cme.medscape.com/viewarticle/502825?rss.

Vogel, G., Buffenstein, A., Minter, K. & Hennessey, A. (1990). Drug effects on REM sleep and on endogenous depression. *Neuropsy. Biobehav. Review*, 14, 49–63.

Zinko, C (2009). That elusive good night's sleep. *SF Chronicle*, 8/17/09. Retrieved August 17, 2009. http://www.sfgate.com/cgi-bin/article.cgi?f=/c/a/2009/08/17/DDNS197N4M.DTL.

Chapter 2

Treatment of Insomnia & Anxiety Disorders

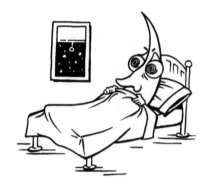

Long before anyone had ever heard of psychiatrists or psychotherapists, people were using alcohol, laudanum, chloral hydrate, kava, and many other substances to help them sleep and to control anxiety. Since the development of barbiturates in the early 20th century, hundreds of drugs to induce sleep and decrease anxiety have been added to the pharmacopeia. The benzodiazepines (BzRAs) were introduced in the 1970s to avoid some of the adverse effects caused by the barbiturates. The newer, widely-used hypnotic agents called "z-compounds" (or non-benzodiazepine receptor agonists), such as zaleplon/Sonata, zolpidem/Ambien, and escitalopram/Lunesta, are in the class of drugs called imidazopyridines. They were developed with the hope of avoiding some of the difficulties that occur with the BzRAs. Ramelteon/Rozerum, a compound which mimics the action of melatonin, is now also on the market.

Due to the high percentages of people with sleep problems, and the assortment of drugs now available, many psychotherapy clients routinely take a wide variety of substances to decrease their anxiety and to help with sleep difficulties. These include prescription drugs, over-the-counter compounds (usually antihistamines), herbs, supplements, and alcoholic beverages.

Manufacturers are continually refining drugs in an attempt to isolate specific effects and to eliminate adverse effects. For example, medical science has long desired a drug that reduces anxiety but does not induce sleep, another that can be used as an anesthetic and not cause a hangover, and still another that prevents seizures and yet would not make patients sleepy. Although researchers are getting closer, as of today the search continues for compounds that completely achieve these goals.

At normal doses, all sedative-hypnotic drugs act on the *limbic* and *cortical* areas in the brain and are CNS depressants. These brain areas play a major role in alertness and sleep. At high doses, some sedative-hypnotic drugs depress the CNS so much that they can induce a coma and possibly cause a fatal *respiratory depression* (sedation of the brain centers that control breathing). BzRAs and the z-compounds will not have this effect unless combined with alcohol.

Sedative-Hypnotic Drugs

Effects on sleep architecture

Sedatives (sometimes called "hypnotic" or "sleep-inducing" drugs) increase total sleep time by about one hour per night. Melatonin-related compounds reduce the time it takes between lying down to the onset of Stage 1 sleep. Taking most sedatives or antianxiety drugs as a sleep aid more frequently than once or twice a week is not usually recommended as it can lead to a decrease in REM sleep. When this happens, there will be a period of REM rebound (the time spent in REM is increased) if the person stops taking the drug. Since REM is a "light" stage of sleep, REM rebound causes a greater number of spontaneous awakenings each night. This will be experienced as an increase in disturbed sleep which will make it even more difficult for the person to stop taking the sedative (Goa & Ward, 1986). (See Fig. 2.1.) Little is known about the effects of long-term use of most hypnotic medications. It is not certain whether, after a few weeks of use, therapeutic effects are maintained, or if the risks of long-term use outweigh the benefits (see below).

As we have seen in Chapter 1, during a normal night of sleep a person progresses from Stage 1 to Delta sleep, back from Delta sleep to Stage 1, and then goes into the first REM period. The first sleep cycle of the night usually takes from 60 to 120 minutes, with an average of about 90 minutes (Kandel & Schwartz, 1981). (See Fig. 1.1.)

Since brain wave patterns in REM sleep are very similar to the wakeful state, one is easily awakened during REM. The reason that people remember their dreams is believed to be due to this similarity of REM to wakefulness. Throughout the night, periods of Delta sleep typically become shorter and periods of REM sleep get longer. As the time spent asleep progresses, people experience more dreams, and a greater percentage of time is spent in the lighter stages of sleep, which in turn leads to more frequent awakenings towards morning (Kandel & Schwartz, 1981).

Tolerance to sedatives

Tolerance (see Appendix E) to the effects of most sedative drugs develops with regular use. Sedatives are most effective when taken only once or twice a week as this will prevent REM rebound. If sedatives are taken intermittently, the patient will have the desired result of fewer awakenings on the nights that the drug is taken. Even with an intermittent dose regimen, Delta sleep, if not eliminated, may be greatly reduced (Dew, et al., 2003). This decrease in Delta sleep can result in not feeling well-rested.

The respiratory centers in the CNS do not habituate quickly to these drugs, whereas the neurons responsible for sleep induction do. This habituation (decrease in effect) leads some people to increase their dose or combine these drugs with alcohol to obtain the desired sedative effect. Since the respiratory centers in the CNS do not habituate at the same rate as the sleep and arousal centers, this behavior can lead to a fatal respiratory depression and must be avoided.

BARBITURATES

Many barbiturates with differing properties have been synthesized. Once widely-prescribed for anxiety and for sleep problems, quite a few are still in use today, primarily as anesthetic agents during surgery and for the treatment of seizure disorders like epilepsy (specifically phenobarbitol).

Barbiturates are classified into several categories as determined by their rates of absorption, distribution, metabolism, and excretion. The shorter-acting compounds are often used under medical supervision as intravenous anesthetics; the longer-acting barbiturates, including phenobarbitol/Luminal, can be used for controlling seizure disorders.

Some barbiturates have proven useful in the treatment of bipolar disorder, particularly for the manic symptoms, and for controlling the aggressive behavior in patients with explosive disorder. Barbiturates are not the first drugs of choice for treatment of these psychiatric disorders, but are tried if other drugs are not effective, are problematic in some way (e.g., cause allergic reactions), or if there are other medical contraindications to the preferred drugs. Barbiturates, taken orally or injected, cause euphoria and can become drugs of abuse.

Enzymatic and *pharmacodynamic tolerances* (see Appendix E) develop with barbiturates. Both types of tolerance contribute to a decrease in their effectiveness.

BENZODIAZEPINES (BZRAS)

The BzRAs were developed with the hope of finding a group of sedative and antianxiety drugs that did not cause physical dependence and had a lower lethality and addictive potential than barbiturates. The attempt was partly successful. The BzRAs reduce anxiety, decrease sleep latency, and have a very low risk of lethality if not combined with other sedatives or with alcohol. BzRAs may also become drugs of abuse for people with a history of addiction.

The BzRAs are a safer treatment for anxiety than barbiturates because they cause less respiratory depression. By acting on GABA (an inhibitory neurotransmitter) (see Appendix C) they also diminish neuronal activity in the areas of the brain associated with emotion: the *septal region*, *amygdala*, hypothalamus, and *hippocampus*. The decrease in neuronal activity in these areas is most likely responsible for reducing anxiety and emotional reactivity as well as for the problems with memory associated with BzRA use (see below).

Medications for Anxiety Disorders

Types of anxiety

Anxiety is classified into two types: somatic and psychological. Somatic anxiety has symptoms such as restlessness, agitation, impatience, hyperactivity, and irritability. These symptoms are associated with high levels of norepinephrine (NE) (Swartz, 2004).

Somatic anxiety may best be treated with beta blockers (e.g., propranolol), BzRAs, anticonvulsants, or antipsychotic drugs. Undertreatment of somatic anxiety may be the cause of the increase in suicidal behaviors seen initially when an SSRI is started for the treatment of anxiety or depression (Swartz, 2004).

Psychological anxiety has symptoms of worry, repetitive thoughts, and dissatisfaction. These are associated with low levels of serotonin and are best treated with SSRIs (Swartz, 2004).

Use of the BzRAs in anxiety disorders

The most appropriate long-term use of BzRAs is for the treatment of Generalized Anxiety Disorder (GAD) and Panic Disorder. GAD is characterized by sustained "free-floating" anxiety, whereas Panic Disorder is characterized by episodes of intense anxiety. Both GAD

Common Benzodiazepines (BzRAs)

- alprazolam/Xanax
- clorazepate/Tranxene
- clonazepam/Klonopin
- chlordiazepoxide/Librium
- diazepam/Valium
- estazolam/ProSom
- flurazepam/Dalmane
- lorazepam/Ativan
- prazepam/Centrax
- oxazepam/Serax
- quazepam/Doral
- temazepam/Restoril
- triazolam/Halcion

Table 2.1

IMPORTANT: Patients should be cautioned never to drink alcohol in combination with BzRAs or any sedative-drug.

and Panic Disorder have a genetic component and aggregate in families (Goa & Ward, 1986).

One disadvantage of taking BzRAs daily for anxiety is that there will be a rebound of anxiety symptoms if the BzRA is discontinued. BzRAs are particularly convenient for anxiety because they can be taken as needed, when the person begins to feel anxious, or when exposed to the specific situation that causes the anxiety. The BzRA usually will take effect and the anxiety will decrease in 15–20 minutes.

When taken for anxiety, the effect of BzRAs on sleep depends on the specific BzRA and the time of day it is taken. If a short or medium-acting BzRA is taken early in the day it will have little effect on sleep. If there is a sleep problem along with the anxiety, a longer-acting BzRA may be most appropriate. However, this may cause problems with daytime sedation and have other adverse effects (see below).

Adverse effects & tolerance to BzRAs

Initial exposure to BzRAs usually causes some impairment in cognitive functioning, in particular difficulty learning (remembering) new information (*anterograde amnesia*). If the BzRA is taken daily, after about two weeks some tolerance to the cognitive impairment and memory difficulties usually develops. Little tolerance will develop to the antianxiety effect or to the impairment of psychomotor performance. This means that even though one may feel mentally clearer, psychomotor skills (e.g., driving) continue to be impaired. Use of BzRAs provides an example of how tolerance to different effects of a drug develops at varying rates and how this can have serious or dangerous consequences.

BzRA addiction & hangover

In general, the more quickly a drug is metabolized, the greater its addictive potential. The shorter-acting BzRAs may be prescribed to help with sleep. In contrast, the slowly-metabolized BzRAs (the ones usually prescribed for anxiety disorders), because of their slower metabolism, may cause a decrease in alertness and hand-eye coordination and may result in falls and a decrease in cognitive ability. This may be particularly problematic for the elderly who generally metabolize drugs more slowly.

Effects of BzRAs on sleep

Tolerance to the sleep-inducing effect of BzRAs develops quickly, leading to a loss in effectiveness for the treatment of insomnia after about two weeks of continuous use (Armitage, et al., 1997). For an optimal sleep-inducing effect, BzRAs should only be taken every three or four days.

Changes in sleep patterns may occur when a sedative is taken on a long-term basis (over two weeks of daily use) (Armitage, et al., 1997). If the sedative is stopped after this point, a period of rebound insomnia will occur and sleep will be more disrupted than it was with the medication or even before the start of the medication. This rebound effect, and the resulting increase in sleep difficulties, is the reason that it is very difficult for most people to stop taking BzRAs for sleep after they have become habituated to them (Kandel & Schwartz, 1981). The newer sleep medications (Ambien, Sonata, Lunesta, Rozerum) were designed with the hope of eliminating this problem (see p. 29).

The graphs in Fig. 2.1 illustrate the effects of older sedatives on sleep architecture:

Graph A: Represents the sleep pattern of someone who woke up twice during the night and was complaining of too many early-morning awakenings. This person wanted medication to help with sleep.

Graph B: Shows the sleep pattern of the same patient just after beginning treatment with a sedative. There are fewer early-morning awakenings, but the periods of deep sleep are already greatly reduced.

Graph C: Represents the patient's sleep patterns after two weeks of taking the sedative on a daily basis. The number of spontaneous awakenings has increased and all periods of deep sleep have been eliminated (Kandel & Schwartz, 1981).

Effects of Sedatives on
Sleep Architecture

Graph A

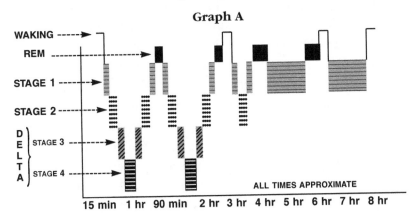

Graph B

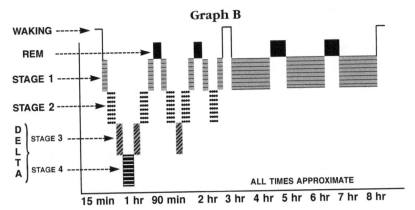

Graph C

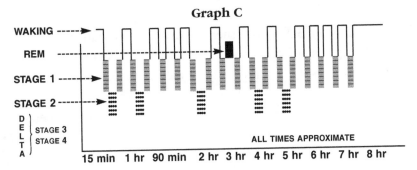

Figure 2.1   (adapted from Kandel & Schwartz 1981)

Effects of BzRAs on memory & pain

BzRAs interfere with the ability to remember new information by inhibiting nerve transmission in the hippocampus. This interference with memory leads to an interesting capacity that the BzRAs have with regard to pain. Although BzRAs have no anesthetic or analgesic effect, they do interfere with the retention of the memory of pain (the anterograde amnesia effect). They are often given along with anesthetic compounds to relax the patient before various medical procedures. This results in patients believing they had little or no pain, but what in fact was diminished was not the pain itself, but the memory of the pain. When an observer is present for a painful procedure in which a BzRA has been given to a patient, the observer may report that the patient reacted as if there had been pain, but the patient, if asked later, will have no memory of it. The question is: if one does not remember pain, how much does it matter whether or not it occurred? (A little like the riddle of the tree falling in the forest: if there's no one there to hear it, does it make any sound?) Somatic psychotherapists believe the memory of the pain is held by the body even if the person cannot consciously recall it.

Most people who take BzRAs on a daily basis will develop a partial tolerance to the memory-impairment effect in about three weeks. If the BzRA is discontinued, memory usually will return to normal after about one week. The memory impairment is a more serious side effect for patients with dementia.

Withdrawal from BzRAs & other sedative-hypnotic drugs

The symptoms of withdrawal from a sedative-hypnotic drug are often the same as the symptoms for which it was originally taken. If the drug has been taken at high dose levels for a long time, withdrawal may lead to more severe symptoms such as confusion, seizures (which can be fatal), hallucinations, and delusions (Chiang & Goldfrank, 1990). Medical supervision is required for the tapering and discontinuance of sedative medications.

When longer-acting forms of drugs are used, withdrawal symptoms can appear several days after the last dose, and may continue for two to three weeks. With shorter-acting forms, the symptoms appear sooner, are more intense, but abate more quickly. The exact length of time it will take for any one person to withdraw from any drug depends on many factors, such as dose, metabolic rate, and personality, and cannot be predicted (Chiang & Goldfrank, 1990).

Frequent symptoms of withdrawal from BzRAs

- irritability
- restlessness
- insomnia
- muscle tension

Other possible symptoms of BzRA withdrawal

- seizures
- blurred vision
- feelings of weakness
- increased blood pressure
- hypersensitivity to light and sound
- nightmares
- rapid heartbeat
- aches and pains

A psychiatrist needs to oversee a slow tapering of the dose both for safety and to ease the symptoms of withdrawal. The usual regimen is to reduce the dose 5% to 10% a day for a week or two. If a patient has been taking a short-acting drug, a longer-acting preparation may be substituted first, then tapered off. The procedure of switching from a shorter-acting to a longer-acting compound usually prevents seizures and lessens discomfort (Chiang & Goldfrank, 1990).

IMPORTANT: The danger of seizures is highest more than one week after the last dose of the sedative.

NON-BENZODIAZEPINE (Z-COMPOUNDS) FOR SLEEP

This class of hypnotic drugs includes eszopiclone/Lunesta, zaleplon/Sonata, and zolpidem/Ambien; these are now widely used for sleep difficulties. Because they are

Imidazopyridines (z-compounds)
• eszopiclone/Lunesta
• zaleplon/Sonata
• zolpidem/Ambien
Table 2.2

metabolized rapidly, there is less drowsiness or drug-hangover the next day. Drugs in this class are already the first-line treatment for insomnia and may eventually replace the BzRAs as a treatment for sleep problems.

In a randomized, double-blind, placebo-controlled study, eszopiclone/Lunesta retained its effectiveness in increasing total sleep time (as assessed by patient questionnaire). In this study, the drug was taken consecutively for as long as six months (Krystal, et al., 2003).

There are recent reports of serious allergic reactions to these drugs and strange behaviors while asleep, like driving, eating, and having sex, for which the person has no memory the next day. The FDA has required that a "black box warning" be placed on the information packets for these drugs.

RAMELTEON

Ramelteon/Rozerum is different from the BzRAs and the z-compounds in that it mimics the action of melatonin and shortens sleep latency. Patients may experience an increase in therapeutic effects over a period of several nights or weeks. This medication is not associated with any cognitive or psychomotor impairment or with strange sleep behaviors. Ramelteon has been shown to have potential for abuse (Neubauer, 2009).

Other Medications for Insomnia

TRAZODONE

Trazodone/Desyrel is a tri-cyclic antidepressant medication that is frequently prescribed as a sleep aid. It is not FDA-approved for this use and there are no placebo-controlled studies to support its use in this way (Wiegand, 2008). There is no risk of abuse with trazodone, and if the sleep problem is due to depression this drug may be an appropriate treatment for both conditions.

ANTIHISTAMINES

Over-the-counter (OTC) sleep aids (e.g., Tylenol PM) usually contain antihistamines, either diphenhydramine/Benadryl, promethazine, or doxylamine. These aid sleep by causing a non-selective blockage of histamine receptors. This blockage of histamine induces sleep by shortening sleep latency (Gengo, et al., 1989). These preparations are usually safe, but there are a wide variety of possible responses. Some people do not get sleepy, and among those who do, some develop a tolerance to the sleep-induction effect quite rapidly, sometimes after taking the drug only once or twice (Richardson, et al., 2002). Some people who experience improved sleep have a drug hangover the next day. This can usually be prevented by taking the antihistamine earlier in the evening (Gengo, et al., 1989). There have also been reports of excessive sedation and weight gain. Selective histamine (H1) antagonists are under development (Stahl, 2008), and it is hoped that these will not have the adverse effects of the non-selective histamine blockers.

Adverse effects of antihistamines

Because they are considered relatively safe, historically antihistamines have been widely used for the treatment of insomnia in children and the elderly. Recent studies indicate that there may be some cognitive impairment in the elderly who use them as a sleep aid (Simons, et al., 1999). Antihistamine use also leads to a suppression of REM sleep and to a period of REM rebound when the drug is discontinued (Gengo, et al., 1989). For some people, antihistamines (when used intermittently) are very effective for sleep problems.

Risk of taking antihistamines during pregnancy

There is some indication that antihistamines may cause birth defects if taken during the first trimester. To decrease risk, it is best that no medications be taken during pregnancy (Miller, 2002).

ACT-078573 (ALMOREXANT)

Almorexant is in Phase III clinical trials in many sites worldwide. It is an *antagonist* (see Appendix D) to orexin, a neurotransmitter that maintains wakefulness (see Chapter 1). The researchers are doing placebo-controlled and comparison-polysomnographic studies to see how the stages of sleep are effected by this drug. The final results are not yet published (Clinical trials.gov, 2009).

Other Medications for Anxiety Disorders

SSRIs

At present, SSRIs (along with cognitive therapy) are generally considered the first choice for treatment of symptoms of anxiety whether the anxiety is due to GAD, OCD, panic disorder, or post-traumatic stress disorder (PTSD). Since the SSRI may take a few weeks to fully take effect, a BzRA is often prescribed for immediate symptom relief. Symptoms of OCD usually require a higher dose of the SSRI and the symptoms may take longer to remit than for the other anxiety disorders.

The SSRIs do not decrease tension. Tension can provoke violent acts such as suicide (Swartz, 2004). More detailed information on SSRIs can be found in Chapter 4.

BUSPIRONE

Buspirone/Buspar does not have muscle-relaxant, sedative, or anticonvulsant effects. It is not structurally similar to the BzRAs or other sedatives. Unlike the BzRAs, it does not bind to the GABA receptors; instead, it binds to 5-HT and DA receptors (Armitage, 1997).

A major advantage of buspirone is that it has a very low risk of lethality if taken by itself. It can be used by people who drink since it does not add to the effects of alcohol or other drugs that depress the CNS. In addition, it does not cause euphoria, so there is little risk of abuse. This drug does not cause impairment of cognitive functioning, memory, or psychomotor skills.

Buspirone seems to be as effective as the BzRAs in the treatment of GAD, and has been found effective for treating depressive symptoms in anxious patients. This is a major advantage over the BzRAs, since the BzRAs may increase symptoms of depression (Armitage, 1997). Buspirone does not decrease muscle tension as do the BzRAs.

Adverse effects of buspirone

The frequency of adverse effects with buspirone is very low. Some people may experience dizziness, headache, nausea, and diarrhea. These symptoms decrease if the person stays on the drug long enough to become habituated (usually one or two weeks). The major drawback with buspirone is that it is designed to be taken on a daily basis, unlike the BzRAs, which are taken as needed.

PROPRANOLOL

The drug propranolol/Inderal was developed for the treatment of high blood pressure and cardiac arrhythmias, for which it is very effective and has few adverse effects. It is in the class of drugs called "beta blockers." This drug is useful for people with panic attacks because it decreases the *enteroceptive* (internally generated) cues of anxiety, specifically rapid heartbeat and increased blood pressure. In people with a history of panic attacks, it often is an internal signal of anxiety, such as rapid heartbeat, that can precipitate an attack.

Although used for panic attacks, propranolol is not FDA-approved as an antianxiety medication; therefore, this is considered an "off label" use. Propranolol should not be used as an antianxiety medication for people with cardiac problems. Serious rebound phenomena can occur if this medication is stopped abruptly. In particular, an increase in cardiac irregularities that can lead to a potentially fatal disruption in heart functioning.

Propranolol does not interfere with memory or psychomotor

performance. For this reason, and because it decreases stage fright, it has become popular with public speakers, musicians, performers, and people taking various licensure examinations. For a person with a specific phobia or a history of substance abuse, propranolol may be the most appropriate drug as an antianxiety medication because it does not produce feelings of euphoria, has no potential for abuse, and can be taken as needed.

Propranolol for PTSD

Recent studies seem to indicate that taking propranolol after a trauma may prevent the development of PTSD (Pitman, et al., 2002). If propranolol is given soon after a trauma, the memories do not seem to be stored in the same way that traumatic memories are usually stored, and therefore PTSD does not develop.

Adverse effects of propranolol

Some of the possible adverse effects of propranolol are:

- nausea
- vomiting
- depression
- a potentially dangerous worsening of asthma

PRAZOSIN FOR PTSD NIGHTMARES

Prazosin is FDA-approved for the treatment of high blood pressure and prostate problems. It has been on the market for many years with no serious long-term adverse effects. Researchers have found it to be helpful for sleep disturbances and nightmares in people with PTSD (Miller, 2008).

Prazosin is not a sedative; it does not induce sleep. The drug seems

Other Drugs for Anxiety and Sedation	
• buspirone/Buspar	• hydroxyzine/Atarax, Vistaril
• clonidine/Catapres	• melatonin
• escitalopram/Lexapro	• paroxetine/Paxil
• diphenhydramine/Benadryl	• propranolol/Inderal
• gabapentin/Neurontin	• sodium oxybate/Xyrem

Table 2.3

to lead to longer and better sleep by blocking NE and increasing REM sleep. Veterans with PTSD taking prazosin reported feeling generally better due to an improvement in their sleep. It has been taken for many years without inducing tolerance or any increase in dose. When the drug is stopped, the nightmares usually return (Miller, 2008).

GLUTAMATE RECEPTOR (mGLU) AGONIST FOR ANXIETY

LY354,740/Eglumegad is a glutamate receptor agonist that reduces neuronal transmission in brain regions involved in anxiety and stress. It is not yet FDA-approved. In a preclinical study, this drug reduced anxiety without causing a sedative effect. It offers advantages over the BzRAs, which cause sedation and memory problems as undesirable side effects. The form of this compound being tested currently is the prodrug LY544,344 which has better bioavailability than LY354,740 (Perkins & Abraham, 2007).

D-CYCLOSERINE (DCS) FOR PHOBIAS

Years of preliminary research have demonstrated that the medication D-cycloserine (DCS) (marketed as a tuberculosis medication under the brand name Seromycin) can boost the effectiveness of therapy in treating a variety of simple phobias. DCS is currently in Phase II clinical trials for phobia treatment. It has been shown to facilitate fear-reduction in social phobia and fear of heights (Ressler, et al., 2004).

DCS appears to work by affecting the NMDA receptor (a type of glutamate receptor) in the amygdala portion of the brain. It is not yet clear if this is its only effect. The drug appears to stimulate the area of the brain that is responsible for unlearning fear responses (Ressler, et al., 2004).

Electrical Stimulation Methods for Anxiety Disorders

DEEP BRAIN STIMULATION (DBS) FOR OCD

In February 2009, the U.S. Food and Drug Adminstration announced approval of Reclaim Deep Brain Stimulation (DBS) Therapy for chronic, severe, obsessive-compulsive disorder (OCD). This procedure involves the implantation of a pulse-generator into the brain of affected individuals.

OCD patients who may be candidates for DBS are adults who have a primary diagnosis of severe OCD, who have had the disease for at least five years, and are referred by their treating psychiatrist. The patients must have refractory OCD as defined by having failed at least three SSRI trials, one of which must have been with clomipramine (at maximum-tolerated dose for an adequate period of time). They must also fail to improve with cognitive-behavior therapy (CBT). The procedure for the implantation of the pulse-generator was found to be relatively safe (Lyons, et al., 2004), although there is always some degree of risk involved with brain surgery.

TRANSCRANIAL MAGNETIC STIMULATION (TMS) FOR PTSD

In a preliminary study, patients were given ten TMS sessions, one per day, each 20 minutes long. Both the patients and their doctors assessed improvement. Depression and anxiety decreased, and some patients also reported improved sleep and a general increase in calmness. After TMS treatment, patients experienced a lessening of PTSD core symptoms. Headache was the only adverse effect noted (Cohen, et al., 2004).

Direct Relevance to Psychotherapy

Clients frequently come into treatment with sleep problems and many are already taking sleep medications and want to stop. If a client is habituated to a sleep medication, medical oversight is necessary for withdrawal.

Sedatives are effective as antiseizure medications because they increase the seizure threshold (i.e., they decrease the likelihood of a seizure by depressing the CNS). Because of this effect, withdrawal from these drugs leads to an increased likelihood of seizures or convulsions which can be fatal. Other disturbing symptoms frequently experienced during sedative withdrawal are agitation, hallucinations, and disorientation. When sedatives are withdrawn, REM rebound occurs, leading to an increase in the symptoms of insomnia. The worsening of the insomnia may last until the withdrawal period is over, which sometimes takes weeks.

It is not unusual for clients who are taking BzRAs for sleep problems to report that their problems have continued despite the drugs and that they have increased their dose hoping to obtain the desired effect of a better night's sleep. Unfortunately, most people do not know that increasing the dose will not, in the long run, improve sleep. Using sleep medications can result in a dangerous cycle of increasing dosage and continued poor sleep. If a client reports these problems, and wants to continue using a sedative, the psychotherapist should recommend an evaluation by a psychiatrist.

Many new drugs are being tested for the treatment of PTSD, and new methods are on trial for the treatment of refractory OCD. The future effectiveness is not yet certain, but there is hope that these difficult-to-treat conditions will be helped with these newer methods of treatment.

References for Chapter 2

Armitage, R., Yonkers, K., Cole, D. & Rush, J. (1997). A multicenter, double-blind comparison of the effects of nefazodone and fluoxetine on sleep architecture and quality of sleep in depressed outpatients. *J. Clinical Psychopharm.*, 17(3), 161-168.

Chiang, W. & Goldfrank, L. (1990). Substance withdrawal. *Emergency Medicine Clinics of North America*, 8(3), 613-631.

Clinical trials. gov. (2009). Almorexant in Adult Subjects With Chronic Primary Insomnia (RESTORA 1), Updated: October 30, 2009, Retrieved December 26, 2009. http://www.clinicaltrials.gov/ct2/show/NCT00608985?term=almorexant&rank=1.

Cohen, H., Kaplan, Z., Kotler, M., Kouperman, I., Moisa, R. & Grisaru, N. (2004). Repetitive-transcranial magnetic stimulation of the right dorsolateral prefrontal cortex in posttraumatic-stress disorder: A double-blind, placebo-controlled study. *Am. J. Psychiatry*, 161, 515-24.

Dew, M., Hoch, C., Buysse, D., Monk, T., Begley, A., Houck, P., Hall, M., Kupfer, D. & Reynolds, C. (2003). Healthy older adults' sleep predicts all-cause mortality at 4 to 19 years of follow up. *Psychosomatic Medicine*, 65, 63-73.

Gengo, F., Gabros, C. & Miller, J. (1989). The pharmacodynamics of diphenhydramine-induced drowsiness and changes mental performance. *Clin. Pharm. Therapeutics*, 45(1), 15-21.

Goa, K. & Ward, A. (1986). Buspirone. A preliminary review of its pharmacological properties as a function of drug level in generalized anxiety. *Drugs*, 32(2), 114-129.

Kandel, E. & Schwartz, J. (1981). *Principles of Neuroscience*. NY, NY: Elsevier North Holland, Inc.

Krystal, A., Walsh, J., Laska, E., Caron, J., Amato, D., Wessel, T. & Roth, T. (2003). Sustained efficacy of eszopiclone over 6 months of nightly treatment: Results of a randomized, double-blind, placebo-controlled study in adults with chronic insomnia. *Sleep*, 26(7), 793-9. Abstract.

Lyons, K., Wilkinson, S., Overman, J., & Pahwa, R. (2004). Surgical and hardware complications of subthalamic stimulation: A series of 160 procedures. *Neurology*, 63, 612-16.

Miller, A. (2002). Diphenhydramine toxicity in a newborn: A case report. *J. Perinatol.*, 20(6), 390-391.

Miller, L. (2008). Prazosin for the treatment of posttraumatic stress disorder sleep disturbances. *Pharmacotherapy*, 28(5), 656-66.

Neubauer, D. (2009). Insomnia: Recent advances in pharmacological management. Retrieved March 22, 2010. http://www.psychiatrictimes.com/sleep disorders/content/article/1145628/1490698

Perkins, E. & Abraham, T. (2007). Pharmacokinetics, metabolism, and excretion of the intestinal peptide transporter 1 (SLC15A1)-targeted prodrug (1S,2S,5R,6S)-2-[(2'S)-(2-amino)propionyl]aminobicyclo[3.1.0.]hexen-2,6-dicarboxylic acid (LY544344) in rats and dogs: Assessment of first-pass bioactivation and dose linearity. *Drug Metabolism and Disposition: The Biological Fate of Chemicals*, 35 (10): 1903-9.

Pitman, R., Sanders, K., Zusman, R., Healy, A., Cheema, F., Lasko, N., Cahill, L. & Orr, S. (2002). Pilot study of secondary prevention of posttraumatic stress disorder with propranolol. *Biological Psychiatry*, 51, 189-192.

Ressler, K., Rothbaum, B., Tannebaum, L., Anderson, P., Graap. K., Zimand, E., Hodges, L. & Davis, M. (2004). Cognitive enhancers as adjuncts to psychotherapy: Use of D-cycloserine in phobic individuals to facilitate extinction of fear. *Arch. of Gen. Psychiatry*, 61, 1136-144.

Richardson, G., Roehrs, T., Rosenthal, L., Koshorek, G. & Roth, T. (2002). Tolerance to daytime sedative effects of H1 antihistamines. *J. Clin. Psychopharm.*, 22(5), 511-515.

Simons, F., Fraser, T., Maher, J., Pillay, N. & Simons, K. (1999). Central nervous system effects of H1-receptor antagonists in the elderly. *Ann. Allergy Asthma Immunol.*, 82(2), 157-160.

Stahl, S. (2008). Selective histamine H1 antagonism: Novel hypnotic and pharmacologic actions challenge classical notions of antihistamines. *CNS Spect.*, 13, 1027-38.

Swartz, C. (2004). Less anxiety but more violence? *Psychiatric Times*, April, 49-50.

Wiegand, M. (2008). Antidepressants for the treatment of insomnia: A suitable approach? *Drugs*, 68, 2411-417.

Chapter 3

Alcohol: Use & Abuse

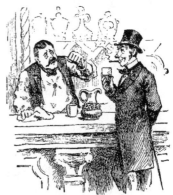

Alcohol (also known as ethanol, grain alcohol, and ethyl alcohol), has a very simple molecular structure that is unlike any other drug discussed in this book. The sedative-hypnotic drugs and alcohol are not chemically related, but their behavioral, physiological, and psychological effects are very similar.

Alcohol, which is one of the most widely-used drugs in western culture, is the intoxicant found in beer, wine, and hard liquor. There is evidence in ancient art and ceramics that alcohol has been used for its intoxicating qualities for at least 6,000 years. Today, between 10.5 million and 14 million Americans suffer from alcoholism, and at least 100,000 deaths each year are associated with alcohol abuse. These fatalities are caused both directly, by damage to the liver and other organs, and indirectly, by automobile or other accidents resulting from alcohol intoxication. Alcohol consumption plays a part in 30%–50% of all traffic fatalities in America (National Institute on Alcohol Abuse & Alcoholism/Databases, 2002). A driver who has had one alcoholic drink is 11 times more likely to be involved in a traffic accident than a driver who has not had any drinks (personal communication, Driving School, 2006).

For most people, moderate use, defined as fewer than two drinks per day, is not a health danger (as long as they do not drive afterward). There is some evidence that one or two glasses of red wine per day may even have some health benefits (Hines, 2000). This research indicates that it is the alcohol, rather than the presence of other compounds (flavinoids), that protects the heart.

In this study, people who metabolize alcohol more slowly had a 30% reduction in heart-attack risk compared to the faster metabolizers. The hypothesis is that the alcohol raises the amount of high-density lipoprotein (HDL) in the blood. The slow metabolizers had more HDL in their blood than the fast metabolizers (Hines, 2000).

The main problem with alcohol use is that many people cannot limit their drinking. The risk of abuse and addiction for these individuals is increased by alcohol's ready availability and low cost.

It is clear that there is a genetic component to alcohol addiction. The chance that the siblings and offspring of alcoholics will become alcoholics themselves is seven times greater than for the general population. Males are particularly at risk. The chance of the average man becoming an alcoholic is 3% to 5%, whereas for the son of an alcoholic the estimates range from 20% to 50%. For women, the chances of becoming alcoholic are between 0.1% and 1%, but for the daughters of alcoholics the risk increases to between 3% and 8% (National Institute on Alcohol Abuse & Alcoholism/Databases, 2002). It is important that close relatives of alcoholics be made aware of their greatly increased risk.

The Process of Intoxication

Alcohol is a small molecule that is soluble in both fat and water. The combination of its small size and solubility make it easy for the alcohol molecule to cross the *blood-brain barrier* (BBB) (see Appendix B, Fig. B1) and other lipid membranes (like the placenta) and for it to get into breast milk. The brain is not protected from high levels of alcohol in the blood stream, so the concentration of alcohol present in the CNS is the same as it is in the rest of the body (Bonner, 1994; Tabakoff & Hoffman, 1993).

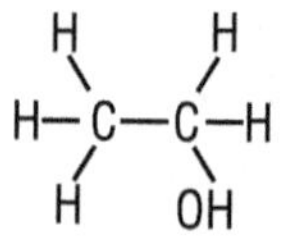

(CH_3CH_2OH)

ethanol

Fig. 3.1

The initial experience after consuming alcohol is usually a feeling of stimulation. This is a result of a disinhibition in the CNS (which takes place at low doses of all sedative-hypnotic compounds). The first part of the brain to be affected is the cortical area; this causes feelings of euphoria accompanied by a decrease in cognitive and judgmental functions.

Various parts of the brain differ in their sensitivity to alcohol. The part that keeps us awake, the *reticular activating system* (RAS), is highly sensitive to alcohol, while the part that controls respiration, the *medulla oblongata*, is the least sensitive area. This differential sensitivity serves as a life-preserver for heavy drinkers, who will usually pass out due to the general depression of the CNS before the level of intoxication is reached where respiration becomes critically impaired. Impairment of respiration requires at least a 0.4% *blood alcohol concentration* (BAC). Estimates of BAC are influenced by many factors such as weight, age, drug use, liver condition, and food and water consumption. The only way to accurately determine BAC is with a blood test or a breathalyzer test.

Effects of Chronic Alcohol Use

The main long-term effects of alcohol use are changes in the hippocampus (which is important in the processes of learning and memory), and liver damage in the form of fat deposits, fibrosis, nodule formations, and cirrhosis of the liver. Although there is evidence that some of the damage to the liver and the brain is due to dietary and vitamin deficiencies, high levels of alcohol consumption also leads to direct damage to the cells of both these vital organs (Beers, et al., 2006).

Pharmacodynamic & metabolic tolerance

Tolerance to alcohol varies widely among individuals. Chronic ingestion leads to both pharmacodynamic and metabolic tolerances (see Appendix E). Pharmacodynamic tolerance results from prolonged exposure of the CNS to alcohol. This exposure causes the cells of the

CNS to become less sensitive to alcohol. When this occurs, a higher BAC is required to attain the desired euphoric effect. Metabolic (enzymatic) tolerance reaches an upper limit and then remains constant. If liver damage occurs, enzymatic tolerance may decrease.

Cross-tolerance

Cross-tolerance can develop between alcohol and other CNS depressants. This means that a person who already has a tolerance to any sedative-hypnotic drug may require a higher dose of alcohol to attain the desired level of intoxication. The cross-tolerance is the result of both pharmacodynamic and metabolic factors. This cross-tolerance does not raise the amount of alcohol that constitutes a lethal dose.

WERNICKE-KORSAKOFF DISEASE

This disease is seen in chronic alcoholics. One cause is a deficiency in vitamin B_1 (Beers, et al., 2006). Alcoholics may get their daily caloric intake from alcohol rather than food, resulting in multiple vitamin deficiencies. Even if drinking continues, many of these symptoms will decrease if B-vitamin supplements are taken. Symptoms include:

- disorientation
- ataxia (dizziness)
- nystagmus (uncontrollable horizontal eye movements) (Beers, et al., 2006)
- apathy
- delirium
- drowsiness

After diagnosis, treatment with B vitamins, administered either intramuscularly or intravenously (for the most rapid effect), is initiated in order to reduce permanent damage to the CNS. Treatment consists of stopping alcohol consumption and continued daily administration of oral B vitamins (Beers, et al., 2006).

ALCOHOL-INDUCED PERSISTING AMNESIC DISORDER

This disorder is characterized by a severe disturbance in the ability to remember recent events. It is found in 80% of patients diagnosed with Wernicke-Korsakoff's disease. Onset is usually after age 40. The disorder may begin insidiously, with no overt symptoms, or may appear suddenly following *delirium tremens* (DTs). The patient has anterograde amnesia for all events that occur after the onset of the illness, and often for events that occurred weeks or months before the onset, as well as *retrograde amnesia* (inability to recall already-learned facts). The patient is unaware of the amnesia, and unknowingly uses *confabulation* (making things up) to cover up the memory deficits.

The anterograde amnesia disorients the sufferer as to time, and although cognitive functioning remains stable, the patient is unable to learn even very simple new information (e.g., remembering the time of day). The person remains alert, is generally cheerful, and seems unaware of the disability. Prognosis for these patients is usually poor (Beers, et al., 2006). Recovery is seen in fewer than 20% of those affected. Even with abstinence, if improvement is not seen in 12 to 18 months after the start of treatment, the disorder is thought to be permanent.

The Computerized Automated Tomography scans (CT), Magnetic Resonance Imaging scans (MRI), and EEG results in these patients can be normal. There are usually hemorrhages in the limbic system of the CNS. Autopsies performed on people with this amnesic disorder show damage to the cells of the hippocampus, parts of the hypothalamus, and the thalamus. The damage is permanent, and is believed to be primarily due to the B-vitamin deficiency (Beers, et al., 2006).

FETAL ALCOHOL SYNDROME (FAS)

FAS is a disease of the newborn that occurs when a woman consumes alcohol during her pregnancy. Symptoms of FAS may occur with as few as two drinks per day; there is evidence of subtle damage to the CNS at even lower levels. The syndrome is seen in the babies of four out of 100 heavy-drinking mothers and is the third-leading cause of birth defects associated with mental retardation (Beers, et al., 2006).

It is not known why the children of some pregnant women who drink get FAS while others do not. Recent research with rats indicates that some of the deficits associated with FAS may be reversed by prenatal treatment with thyroid hormone (Wilcoxon, et al., 2005). The severity of the FAS is proportional to the amount of alcohol consumed. Defects include:

- low birth weight
- cardiovascular defects
- joint and limb abnormalities
- abnormalities in facial structure
- mental retardation (can be quite severe)
- microcephaly (infant's brain is underdeveloped) (Waterson & Murray-Lyon, 1990).

WARNING: No completely safe level of alcohol use during pregnancy has been determined (Waterson & Murray-Lyon, 1990).

Withdrawal from Alcohol

Withdrawal symptoms usually begin 24 to 48 hours after the last drink, although they may not appear for up to three weeks. They can even begin during a period of high alcohol intake if there is a decrease from the usual amount of alcohol consumed (Bonner, 1994). Many in-patient programs use BzRAs or anticonvulsants to ease the symptoms of alcohol withdrawal and to decrease the risk of seizures, which can be fatal even when a patient is hospitalized for detox. When BzRAs are used, the patient is first taken off the alcohol and then slowly tapered off the BzRA. Mild symptoms of withdrawal may include:

- shaking
- sweating
- anxiety
- anorexia
- vomiting
- abdominal cramps

Sleep disturbance is frequent during withdrawal. Typical changes are as follows: increased sleep latency (it takes longer to fall asleep), increased REM sleep (more dreaming), decreased Stage 3 and 4 sleep (more time in lighter stages of sleep). The experience of insomnia can last two weeks or more (see Chapter 1). In more serious cases of withdrawal, auditory and visual hallucinations and paranoid delusions are sometimes present (Chiang & Goldfrank, 1990).

DELIRIUM TREMENS (DTs)

The severe alcohol withdrawal syndrome is known as delirium tremens (DTs) and is seen in up to 10 % of patients in detox. DTs begin with anxiety attacks, confusion, poor sleep, marked sweating, and profound depression. Increases in pulse rate and body temperature parallel the progress of the delirium. The acute period generally lasts from two to ten days, but is sometimes more prolonged (Beers, et al., 2006).

Grand mal seizures occur in 23% to 33% of patients during withdrawal. Three percent of these reach "status epilepticus." This usually occur in patients with a history of a seizure disorder. The mortality rate for this is 1% if the person is treated for the seizure and can reach 15% with no treatment. Death occurs due to an "autonomic storm," a process where the autonomic nervous system is overactive and not able to regulate the life-sustaining processes in the body (Murray & Berger, 1997).

Epilepsy & alcohol withdrawal

When chronic alcohol use is stopped, the CNS becomes hyperexcitable which increases the risk of seizures. Although the period of hyperexcitability can last for several days, the seizure risk peaks within eight to ten hours after the last dose of alcohol. This CNS hyperexcitability is particularly dangerous for people with epilepsy (see above) as they are already at an increased risk for seizures. Anyone with a seizure disorder who has become addicted to alcohol must be monitored very closely during withdrawal. Grand mal seizures may develop within 48 hours after the last drink (Chiang & Goldfrank, 1990).

It has been demonstrated that divalproex sodium/Depakote, a drug used to control seizures, can lessen symptoms during alcohol withdrawal (Reoux, et al., 2001). Use of divalproex sodium would eliminate the need for BzRAs for people who have moderately severe symptoms of alcohol withdrawal. Divalproex has its own side effects (see Chapter 5), so there are pros and cons to using it instead of a BzRA. Most people working in the field prefer using the BzRAs to help with withdrawal (personal communication Jose Maldonato, MD. October 18, 2008).

WARNING: The withdrawal process from alcohol can be fatal even under medical supervision (Chiang & Goldfrank, 1990).

Pharmacological Aids for Abstinence

Disulfiram

The drug disulfiram/Antabuse is sometimes prescribed as a deterrent to alcohol consumption. Taking disulfiram and then drinking alcohol may have unpleasant and possibly fatal consequences. Disulfiram interacts with anything that contains alcohol as well as with many other medications. Any exposure to alcohol, even in small amounts, may cause symptoms of illness. There can be a risk to health if disulfiram is taken when other medical conditions are present (Beers, et al., 2006). (See Appendix D, Fig. D1, for the action of disulfiram on alcohol metabolism.)

The theory behind the use of disulfiram is that a patient's fear of experiencing the unpleasant effects that result from combining disulfiram and alcohol will discourage drinking. In general, taking disulfiram without some form of psychotherapy is not very effective. Some people drink while taking disulfiram and become ill, others stop taking disulfiram rather than not drink. The lack of success of disulfiram in decreasing alcoholism illustrates that punishment is not the optimal method for changing behavior (Carpenter, 2001).

Naltrexone for alcoholism

Studies have shown promising results using the opioid antagonist naltrexone/Vivitrol (extended-release form, lasts for one month) in the treatment of alcoholism (Kranzler, et al., 2009). (See Appendix D for an explanation of the concepts of agonist and antagonist).

Naltrexone was originally developed to treat the cravings

experienced by diacetylmorphine (heroin) addicts during withdrawal (see pp. 151–154). It binds to CNS opioid receptors without producing any sense of euphoria. By preventing the alcohol molecule from binding to the opioid receptors, the rewarding effects are diminished, and the cravings for alcohol are decreased. This makes it easier for someone who has relapsed into drinking to return to abstinence. Behavioral therapy alone reduces relapses to 50%. Relapses are reduced to 20% when patients are treated with the combination of behavioral therapy and naltrexone therapy (Carpenter, 2001).

Calcium acetylhomotaurinate

Calcium acetylhomotaurinate/acamprosate/Campral is approved by the FDA for the treatment of alcoholism. Research on its effectiveness is somewhat equivocal (Bender, 2008). Its chemical structure is similar to the amino acids taurine and GABA. It stimulates the inhibitory actions of GABA while acting as an antagonist against the excitatory effects of glutamate. This combination seems to ease the discomfort of abstinence (Carpenter, 2001). Studies indicate that twice as many people remain abstinent from alcohol while taking calcium acetylhomotaurinate as those not taking any drug and that the rates of abstinence increase the longer the treatment with acamprosate continues (Schuckit, 1997; Tempesta, et al., 2000). Even those patients who did relapse while taking acamprosate had fewer drinks during each relapse (Mason, 2001).

Topiramate

A large (370 subjects) Phase II clinical trial on the antiseizure drug topiramate/Topamax for reducing cravings in alcohol-dependent individuals has recently been completed (Clinical Trials, 2008). The results of this trial are not yet published. In a small, industry-supported study, topiramate was found to be effective in reducing cravings and signs of anxiety in alcohol-dependent individuals (using the definition for dependence found in the *Diagnostic and Statistical Manual* (DSM). The researchers (Johnson, et al., 2003) believe topiramate inhibits the release of DA and that it is through this mechanism that cravings are decreased. Subjects reported that the taste of alcohol was changed while taking topiramate.

Baclofen for alcohol withdrawal

Researchers (Lyon, et al., 2009) are investigating the use of baclofen (a drug used to treat muscle spasms in multiple sclerosis) to ease the symptoms of alcohol withdrawal. The goal is to use lower doses of BzRAs during withdrawal and to achieve the long-term effect of reduced cravings for alcohol.

LY 686017: A neurokinin receptor antagonist

LY 686017 is an investigational drug (George, et al., 2008) that was given to a sample of detoxified alcohol inpatients who had high anxiety scores. LY 686017 works as an antagonist at the substance P neurokinin 1-receptor (NK1R). Cravings were decreased in patients receiving this compound. If proven to be safe and effective, this drug may open up a new mechanism for decreasing cravings in a particular population of recovering alcoholics.

Ketamine psychedelic psychotherapy

There is now a clinic in Tampa Bay, Florida offering ketamine-facilitated psychotherapy (see p. 179) for the treatment of alcohol and drug addiction. The treatment is based on findings by Krupitsky & Grinenko (1997). These researchers found a considerable increase in efficacy of standard alcoholism treatment when it was supplemented by ketamine psychedelic therapy (KPT). Total abstinence for more than one year was observed in 73 out of 111 (65.8%) alcoholic patients in the KPT group, compared to 24% (24 out of 100 patients) of the conventional treatment control group.

Direct Relevance to Psychotherapy

For a variety of therapeutic and practical reasons, it is not advisable for the psychotherapist to attempt to assess the client's level of alcohol use or dependency. If a client wants to stop drinking, the safest way to proceed is to recommend that withdrawal be done under medical supervision. No one can predict the severity of the withdrawal reaction for any individual. There may also be medical conditions present which could complicate and further increase the dangers during the withdrawal process. The best and safest way to support your client during withdrawal is to recommend a consultation with a psychiatrist or a family-practice physician who will supervise the process and provide whatever medical oversight may be needed.

Most therapists believe that alcohol addiction is best treated using a combination of individual psychotherapy and group support. The experience of a group of peers already in recovery provides patients with a new supportive environment where people are not using alcohol. When a person stops drinking, there is great benefit in attending a peer-support group like the 12-step program developed by Alcoholics Anonymous. As always, the best course of treatment must be determined on an individual basis. In some cases, treatment needs to be more behavioral, while in other cases, long-term psychodynamic therapy may be most appropriate.

For clients who desire or require them, there are many new and very helpful and effective medications that ease withdrawal and support and facilitate abstinence. Regardless of additional methods, continuing in individual psychotherapy is highly recommended (Carpenter, 2001), particularly during the early stages of recovery (De Angelis, 2001).

After the initial phase of breaking through the patient's denial, continued confrontation may not be the most effective means of therapy since this may alienate the client and undermine the therapeutic alliance. Therapy can only be effective if the client is being honest with the therapist. If a client fears the therapist's disapproval, the likely result will be that the client will not tell the therapist about the "non-therapeutic" behavior.

Individual psychotherapy is not enough for recovery. It is essential that the client maintain a constant base of support for sobriety (therapy, 12-step meetings, family, friends, church), while developing new habits as a sober person. Depending on the individual, the process of recovery can, and often does, take many years, and there are usually many "slips" before lasting sobriety is achieved.

References for Chapter 3

Beers, M., Porter, R., Jones, T., Kaplan, J. & Berkwits, M. (2006). *The Merck Manual of Diagnosis and Therapy.* 18th Edition. New Jersey: Merck Research Laboratories.

Bender, K. (2008). Alcoholism treatments exert extended effect. *Psychiatric Times,* XXV, (6), 1, 8-9.

Bonner, A. (1994). Biological mechanisms of alcohol dependence. *Current Opinion in Psychiatry,* 7, 262–268.

Carpenter, S. (2001). Mixing medication and psychosocial therapy for alcoholism. *Monitor on Psychology,* June, 36–37.

Chiang, W. & Goldfrank, L. (1990). Substance withdrawal. *Emergency Medicine Clinics of North America,* 8(3), 613–631.

clinicaltrials.gov/show/NCT00210925. Retrieved December 27, 2009. An Efficacy and Safety Study of Topiramate in the Treatment of Alcohol Dependence (2008).

De Angelis, T. (2001). Today's tried-and-true treatments. *Monitor on Psychology,* June, 48–50.

George, T., Gilman, J., Hersh, J., Thorsell, A., Herion, D., Geyer, C., Peng, X., Kielbasa, W., Rawlings, R., Brandt, J., Gehlert, D., Tauscher, J., Hunt, S., Hommer, D. & Helig, M. (2008). Neurokinin 1 receptor antagonism as a possible therapy for alcoholism. *Science,* 319, 1536-539.

Hines, L. (2000). Alcohol protects the heart. *Science News,* 158, 283.

Johnson, B., Ait-Daoud, N., Bowsen, C., Di Clemente, C., Roache, J. & Lawson, K. (2003). Oral topiramate for treatment of alcohol dependence: A randomized controlled trial. *Lancet,* 361, 1677–685.

Kranzler, H., Tennen, H., Armeli, S., Chan, G., Covault, J., Arias, A. & Oncken, C. (2009). Targeted naltrexone for problem drinkers. *J. Clin. Psychopharm.,* 29(4), 350-57.

Krupitsky, E. & Grinenko, A. (1997). Ketamine psychedelic therapy (KPT): A review of the results of ten years of research. *J. Psychoactive Drugs,* 29(2), 165-83.

Lyon, J., Khan, R., Gessert, C. & Larson, P. (2009). Treating alcohol withdrawal with oral baclofen: A randomized, double-blind, placebo-controlled trial. SMDC Health System Thirteenth Annual Minnesota Health Services Research Conference. St. Paul Campus, University of Minnesota.

Mason, B. (2001). Treatment of alcohol-dependent outpatients with acamprosate: A clinical review. *J. Clin. Psychiatry,* 62(Suppl. 20), 42-48.

Murray, T. & Berger, A. (1997). Alcohol withdrawal. *Va. Med. Q.*, 124(3), 184-7, 189.

National Institute on Alcohol Abuse & Alcoholism/Databases. (2002). Retrieved from www.niaaa.nih.gov/databases.

Reoux J., Saxon, A., Malte, C., Sloan, K. & Baer, J. (2001). Divalproex sodium alcohol withdrawal: A randomized double-blind placebo controlled clinical trial. *Alcoho. Clin. Exp. Res.*, 25, 1324–1329.

Schuckit, M. (1997). Science, medicine, and the future: Substance use disorders. *BMJ*, 314, 1605–1608.

Tabakoff, B. & Hoffman, P. (1993). The neurochemistry of alcohol. *Current Opinion in Psychiatry*, 6, 388–394.

Tempesta, E., Janiri, L. & Bignamini, A. (2000). Acamprosate and relapse prevention in the treatment of alcohol dependence: A placebo controlled study. *Alcohol Alcoholism*, 35(2), 202–229.

Waterson, E. & Murray-Lyon, I. (1990). Preventing alcohol-related birth damage: A review. *Social Science and Medicine*, 30, 349–364.

Wilcoxon, J., Kuo, A., Disterhoft, J. & Redei, E. (2005). Behavioral deficits associated with fetal alcohol exposure are reversed by prenatal thyroid hormone treatment: A role for maternal thyroid deficiency in FAE. *Molecular Psychiatry*, 10, 961-71.

Chapter 4

Treatment of Depressive Disorders

For those who have dwelt in depression's dark wood and known its inexplicable agony, their return from the abyss is not unlike the ascent of the poet, trudging upward and upward out of hell's black depths and at last emerging into what he saw as the "shining world."

William Styron

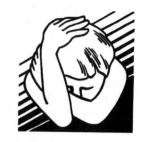

The word "depression" is used in psychology to express a complex phenomenon that has a wide variety of causes as well as symptoms. There are instances when psychotherapy alone can lead to alleviation of symptoms, while at other times the use of antidepressant medication may be both appropriate and necessary to supplement the psychotherapy.

Two common reasons for considering the use of medication as part of the treatment of depression are to facilitate the psychotherapeutic process and to prevent a potential suicide. In addition, a study (Sheline, et al., 1996) has found that recurrent depression has a neurodegenerative component. The structure and function of brain cells in chronically depressed patients are disrupted and nerve-cell connections are destroyed, eventually leading to a decline in cognitive functioning. The rate of recovery appears to decrease when depression becomes chronic (Keller, et al., 1992).

Regardless of the specific cause and type of depression, a commonality in the symptoms and syndromes suggests involvement of the hypothalamus. This part of the brain is responsible for many of the body's regulatory processes such as appetite and the ability to sleep, as well as the ability to experience pleasure. Many of these processes are frequently altered during depression.

If left untreated with either psychotherapy and/or medication, a first episode of depression can last from four to twelve months or longer (the average length being five months). Some typical symptoms are: a pervasive *dysphoric* (unpleasant) mood, a generalized loss of energy, and a state often described by clients as a loss of the ability to experience pleasure (*anhedonia*).

Evidence for a genetic predisposition

Several factors influence one's chances of developing depression. Studies of twins lend strong support to a genetic component. In monozygotic (identical) twins reared together, the concordance rate for depression is 69%, while for fraternal twins the rate is 13%. The concordance rate of identical twins reared apart is 40% to 60% (Kendler & Prescott, 1999). Since the concordance rate is not 100%, the presence of factors other than genetics must also influence the development of depression.

Assessment & Symptoms of Depression

Both the symptoms and the etiology of each client's depression must be considered to determine the most appropriate treatment. Even though the symptoms by themselves tell us little about the cause of a patient's depression, the type of symptoms can help the psychotherapist make more effective interventions. A *DSM* diagnosis of depression requires the presence of the following symptoms:

- loss of energy
- decreased sex drive
- difficulty concentrating
- diminished or increased appetite
- guilty, pessimistic, and suicidal thoughts
- disturbed sleep (usually insomnia with early morning awakening)
- psychomotor agitation or psychomotor retardation

Other common symptoms are a slowing of PSNS functions, such as constipation and decreased salivation. Symptoms are usually worse in the morning, and many people report that towards evening they feel "almost normal." More than 11 million people in the U.S. alone (about 4% of the population) are affected by depression (National Institute of Mental Health {NIMH}, 2003).

> **Vegetative symptoms:** These symptoms strongly suggest a biological component or etiology. Vegetative symptoms typically are:
>
> - weight loss or gain
> - unreactive mood
> - early morning awakening or hypersomnia (sleeping many hours)
> - anhedonia
> - constipation
>
> **Cognitive symptoms:** These symptoms indicate negative thought patterns:
>
> - feelings of helplessness
> - difficulty concentrating
> - feelings of guilt
> - decreased self-esteem
>
> **Behavioral symptoms:** This cluster of symptoms reflects a change in normal behavior patterns such as:
>
> - psychomotor retardation (pronounced slowness or lack of movement)
> - psychomotor agitation (jittery and increased movement)

As a group, patients with vegetative symptoms are the most likely to need medication for optimal improvement. A person with cognitive symptoms might benefit more from cognitive interventions, or if there are many behavioral symptoms, behavioral interventions might be most effective. A combination of Cognitive Behavioral Therapy (CBT) and medication is believed to be the most effective combination for treatment of depression.

If not properly diagnosed and treated, depression can have serious, long-term consequences. Personal relationships and employment can suffer greatly due to lack of motivation and lack of enjoyment in life. The risks of a negative outcome, such as cognitive losses, damaged relationships, and non-response to treatment with medication, are increased when a depression is left untreated for many months (Keller, et al., 1992; Sheline, 1996; Oquendo, et al., 1999).

Subtypes of Depression

It can be useful to classify depression into subtypes according to a person's response to various psychoactive medications. These categories do not correspond directly to *DSM* diagnostic categories because in the *DSM* patients are grouped primarily by response to medication.

Psychotic or Delusional Depression

In a psychotic or delusional depression, there is a preponderance of vegetative symptoms with the addition of delusions. The delusions are mood-congruent and are usually paranoid in nature. Decreased REM latency (see Chapter 1) is often present. This type of depression responds best to antipsychotic medication. After psychotic symptoms clear, the patient needs to be reevaluated for further appropriate interventions.

Recurrent Unipolar Depression

This is the most common type of depression (Greden, 2001). It is generally believed to be due to a biochemical imbalance. It is the type which is most responsive to pharmacological treatment. Currently, the first drug of choice is one of the SSRIs. These patients generally have a stable lifestyle, do not have a family history of alcoholism, and do not show signs of a personality disorder. They usually say that they do not know why they are depressed; there is no clear precipitating incident. Recovery rates for this group are good; about 75% improve on SSRIs or *heterocyclic antidepressants* (HCAs), and about 70% respond to *electroconvulsive therapy* (ECT). These patients also have the highest risk of relapse (Avery & Lubrano, 1979; Fink, 2001; Keller, et al., 1992).

DEPRESSIVE SPECTRUM DISORDER

These patients usually present with a chaotic lifestyle which is punctuated by disruptions such as divorce, violence, sexual problems, difficulties with employment, and a family history of alcoholism. Disturbances in eating and sleeping are also frequent. Statistically, they have fewer previous episodes of depression than the unipolar group, and they are somewhat less responsive to SSRIs and HCAs. About 50% are helped by medication.

ATYPICAL DEPRESSION

There are two types of atypical depression: the vegetative type, with symptoms of *hypersomnia* (oversleeping) and *hyperphagia* (compulsive overeating), and the anxiety type, with symptoms of anxiety, restlessness, and nervousness. Panic attacks and phobias may also be present in the anxiety type (Fox-Aarons, et al., 1985).

People in this group retain emotional reactivity and do not display the flatness of affect often seen with depression. They are frequently hypersensitive to criticism, hyperreactive to rejection, and often have GI symptoms. People in this group may respond preferentially to *monoamine oxidase inhibitors* (MAOIs) (Fox-Aarons, et al., 1985). In current practice, an SSRI is usually tried first because the side effects are more benign and patients do not have to modify their eating habits (as is necessitated with higher doses of MAOIs). If the depression is not treated effectively, these people may eventually develop unipolar depression (Fox-Aarons, 1985).

Note: There is no correlation between "atypical" depression and the use of "atypical" antidepressant drugs.

BIPOLAR DISORDER (See Chapter 5 for a detailed discussion.)

This is usually considered to be primarily a biological disorder. It is now clear that the first treatment of choice is lithium. If this is not sufficient, lamotrigine/Lamictal, or thyroid hormone, may be added to the patient's regimen to treat the depressive part of the disorder.

Antidepressant Medications by Type

In general, the different types of antidepressant medications are equally effective depending on the type of depression (see above). The choice of the specific drug is usually made based upon side-effect profile, prior history of good results, and safety. The initial effect of any antidepressant may be one of calming; even after only one or two days on medication the patient may begin to feel somewhat better. On the other hand, it can be as many as eight to ten weeks before the full effect of the medication is attained. Antidepressant medications are effective for decreasing a moderately-severe depression in about two-thirds of patients (Oquendo, et al., 1999).

SELECTIVE SEROTONIN REUPTAKE INHIBITORS (SSRIs)

SSRIs facilitate improvement in mood, decrease hyperreactivity and hypersensitivity, and help to relieve disruptions in sleeping and eating. Prior to the development of the SSRIs, the major difficulty in treating depression with medication was the dangerous combination of the high risk of suicide in this group of patients coupled with the lethality of the available drugs (TCAs and HCAs, see p. 64) (Lane, et al., 1995).

Because of their low level of lethality, SSRIs have made pharmacological intervention much less risky, which has led to the extensive use of this group of drugs for mild to moderate depression.

As of August 2009, an estimated 40 million people had been treated with just one type of SSRI (Prozac), with millions more taking others. This widespread use of SSRIs has contributed to the growing

---

Common SSRIs

- citalopram/Celexa
- escitalopram/Lexapro
- fluvoxamine/Luvox
- fluoxetine/Prozac
- paroxetine/Paxil
- sertraline/Zoloft
- venlafaxine/Effexor
  (an SNRI at higher doses)

Table 4.1

need for psychotherapists to understand the use and misuse of these medications. At present, it is common for every therapy practice to have clients on some type of antidepressant medication, most typically one of the SSRIs.

Adverse effects of SSRIs

When starting SSRIs many people may experience:
- hyperactive reflexes
- GI disturbances
- restlessness
- irritability
- decrease in sexual desire
- decreased ability to achieve orgasm
- disturbances in sleep patterns and dreams
- GI bleeding when combined with anti-inflammatory drugs (Mort, et al., 2006)

After a period of adjustment of one or two weeks, many of the initial adverse effects abate (Lane, et al., 1995).

Sexual dysfunction

It is estimated that between 30% and 70% of patients on SSRIs experience some degree of sexual dysfunction (Clayton, et al., 2002). The disturbance in sexual function seems to be the adverse effect most resistant to habituation, and the one that causes the most people to decide to discontinue treatment with SSRIs. Sexual response returns to normal when the SSRI is discontinued. Studies show that sildenafil/Viagra may be effective for both men and women as a treatment for the sexual dysfunction caused by SSRI use (Clayton, et al., 2002; Nurnberg, et al., 1999).

Some psychiatrists believe this problem may be lessened by skipping one day of medication (and planning to have sex on that day). Manufacturers claim the newer SSRIs (citalopram/Celexa, venlafaxine/Effexor, escitalopram/Lexapro) have fewer adverse effects, particularly with regard to sexual dysfunction. It has also been noted that SSRIs can be helpful for premature ejaculation since they delay orgasm (Arafa & Shamloul, 2007).

Movement disorders

Evidence suggests that SSRIs can cause movement disorders similar to those seen in the *extrapyramidal syndrome* (EPS) caused by antipsychotic medications (Diler, et al., 2002). (See Chapter 7.)

Black box warning

The FDA issued a health advisory in March, 2004, urging close monitoring of adults and children taking antidepressants and asked manufacturers to include stronger warnings on the labels. Many drugs currently on the market have not been tested or approved for use in children, in the geriatric population, or in pregnant women.

SSRIs and pregnancy

All antidepressants diffuse across the placenta. No psychotropic drug has yet been approved by the FDA for use during pregnancy. The FDA and Wyeth Pharmaceuticals have announced revised label warnings stating that neonates exposed to venlafaxine (as well as other SSRIs and SNRIs) late in the third trimester of pregnancy have developed complications requiring prolonged hospitalizations, respiratory support, and tube feeding.

In a large study, SSRIs were not associated with major malformations overall but were significantly associated with cardiac septal defects, particularly if taken in the first trimester of pregnancy (Pedersen, et al., 2009). All of the antidepressant drugs (including SSRIs) have been associated with higher rates of spontaneous abortion.

SSRIs and increased suicide risk

The controversy about the use of SSRIs in teens has not been definitively resolved. Different types of studies lead to different interpretations of results. The debate has been extended to include increased risk of suicidal thoughts and behaviors for adults.

At present, fluoxetine/Prozac is the only SSRI approved for the treatment of depression in children and adolescents. Research (Hall, et al., 2003) indicates that the medication lessens their risk.

There is no way to differentiate which teens are at risk because of the drug from those who are at risk from their depression without medication (Carey, 2004). Other studies (Nemeroff, et al., 2007) indicate that the decrease in SSRI prescriptions following the FDA warning has led to an increase in completed suicides in youths (Kalikow, 2008).

One analysis of the records of 160,000 adults and children showed that the risk of suicide was highest during the first three or four weeks of treatment. As of now, no research has indicated any significant differences between the different drugs or quantified the risks of stopping the antidepressants (Martinez, et al., 2005).

Results of many large studies are contradictory. One meta-analysis looked at data from many studies; a total of over 200,000 subjects in three reviews (Gibbons, et al., 2007). Suicide attempts occurred in less than 0.5 percent of the subjects. One study looked at over 40,000 people and found no evidence that SSRIs increased the rate of suicide (Martinez, et al., 2005). Another compared patients on SSRIs and those taking placebos or getting other forms of therapy. This study found that the rate of suicide attempts was twice as high in the group taking SSRIs (Fergusson, et al., 2005). This may only indicate that those taking medication had more serious depressions. Research on this topic continues.

Toxic serotonin syndrome (TSS)

Toxic serotonin syndrome is a potentially life-threatening complication caused by drugs that enhance serotonin activity in the CNS. It is usually caused by the use of more than one serotonin-enhancing drug at the same time. TSS may be hard to recognize because of the varied and nonspecific nature of its clinical features. Symptoms of TSS are alterations in:

- behavior (agitation, restlessness)
- cognition (disorientation, confusion)
- neuromuscular activity (cramping, hyperactive reflexes, muscle spasms)

- autonomic nervous system function (fever, shivering, sweating, diarrhea)(Lane & Baldwin, 1997)

It is important that both the therapist and the client be aware of these symptoms, particularly if the client is using more than one serotonin-enhancing drug (e.g., taking MDMA/"ecstasy" while using an SSRI). If these symptoms are seen, immediate referral to a physician is essential so that a medical evaluation and any necessary treatment can be instituted. TSS can be fatal if not treated promptly (Lane & Baldwin, 1997).

SEROTONIN NOREPINEPHRINE REUPTAKE INHIBITORS (SNRIS)

SNRIs are antidepressants that affect both the NE and 5-HT systems; these are being called "dual action" antidepressants. This is a valuable characteristic because some depressions respond better to medications

Common SNRIs
• duloxetine/Cymbalta
• venlafaxine/Effexor
Table 4.2

that primarily affect the NE system, while others respond better to those that primarily affect the 5-HT system.

Venlafaxine/Effexor, one of the SSRIs, has been shown to also inhibit reuptake of NE (Manfredonia, 1997). The NE response for venlafaxine is dose-dependent, with NE more affected by higher doses (over 150 mg/day) (Manfredonia, 1997). Patients who do not respond to other SSRIs may respond to venlafaxine, thus obtaining the benefits of its action on NE and 5-HT while taking a medication (venlafaxine) which does not have the adverse effects and risks inherent in the tricyclic and heterocyclic antidepressants.

Another SNRI, duloxetine/Cymbalta, is FDA-approved for both depression and GAD. This drug exerts NE and 5-HT reuptake inhibition throughout its dose range. It is being advertised as helping with the "pain" of depression. There is evidence that it helps with many kinds of pain, not just pain related to depression (Perahia, et al., 2006). Caution should be exercised when duloxetine is taken as it interacts with many other drugs (Goldstein, et al., 2004).

TRICYCLIC & HETEROCYCLIC ANTIDEPRESSANTS (TCAs & HCAs)

Before the advent of the SSRIs, the first choice of medication for depression was either a TCA or an HCA. HCAs were developed to improve on efficacy and decrease the adverse effects seen with TCAs. While no longer the drugs of first choice, TCAs and HCAs are still used, either for patients already on them who are having positive results with minimal adverse effects, or for patients who do not have an adequate response to SSRIs or SNRIs. There is evidence that more severe depressions respond preferentially to HCAs (Guelfi, et al., 2001).

Since TCAs and HCAs have been on the market for many years, an extensive body of research exists as to their efficacy. Without either medication or psychotherapy, 25% of people with mild to moderate depression will experience a remission of symptoms; with a placebo, the rate is 40%; and with TCAs or HCAs the rate of remission is 70%.

Adverse effects of TCAs & HCAs

Some adverse effects are common when starting on TCAs or HCAs. Most frequently seen are:

- initial sedation
- psychomotor slowing
- dry mouth
- difficulty concentrating
- constipation
- muscle twitching
- possible lowering of the seizure threshold
- increased risk of a manic episode (can indicate too high a dose or bipolar disorder)

Lethality of TCAs & HCAs

This group of medications can be cardiotoxic, particularly for

---

Common TCAs & HCAs
(Tricyclic & Heterocyclic Antidepressants)

- amitriptyline/Elavil
- imipramine/Tofranil
- clomipramine/Anafranil
- maprotiline/Ludiomil
- desipramine/Norpramin
- nortriptyline/Aventyl, Pamelor
- doxepin/Sinequan, Adapin
- protriptyline/Vivactil

Table 4.3

patients with heart disease. In high doses, they can cause a disruption in electrical conduction of the heart (Roose, et al., 1987). One week's worth of medication, if taken all at once, can be fatal.

It is very dangerous to give the group of patients at greatest risk for suicide a drug that can easily be used for this. Before the availability of the SSRIs and SNRIs, the risk of providing a patient with the means to commit suicide was the major concern for psychiatrists prescribing antidepressant medication. If TCAs or HCAs are being used, and the risk of suicide is high, taking precautionary measures, such as putting a family member in charge of dispensing medication, or having the person hospitalized so medication is dispensed by staff, is essential.

MONOAMINE OXIDASE INHIBITORS (MAOIS)

The first monoamine oxidase inhibitor (MAOI) found to be effective as an antidepressant was iproniazid, a drug that was being tested for the treatment of tuberculosis. During clinical trials, some patients who were depressed reported an unexpected elevation in mood. Iproniazid was then tested on patients specifically diagnosed with depression and found to be effective in alleviating their symptoms.

Most MAOIs work by irreversibly binding to the MAO enzyme and thus preventing the breakdown of the monoamines, DA, NE and 5-HT. The net result of this process is an increase in monoamines in the body. The presence of very large amounts of NE can lead to a *hypertensive crisis* (a dangerous elevation of blood pressure). For this reason, if MAOIs are to be used safely at higher doses, diet must be restricted to prevent a hypertensive crisis. This can be problematic, since it is very difficult for most people to change their eating habits. Although atypical depression responds preferentially to MAOIs, these drugs are not frequently prescribed due to the fear of serious side effects if appropriate restrictions are not followed (see below).

Usually, MAOIs are tried when a patient does not respond to SSRIs, SNRIs, HCAs or TCAs. A transdermal form of MAOI, selegiline/Emsam is now available. Dietary restrictions are not required at the usual dose of Emsam. (See transdermal selegiline, below.)

Dietary restrictions with MAOIs

Tyramine, an amino acid, is a precursor for NE. Consuming foods that contain large amounts of tyramine leads to an increase in the synthesis of NE, which could lead to a hypertensive crisis. Hence the need for a restricted diet. Some food additives also increase the synthesis of NE. A text on nutrition can be consulted for a complete list of the tyramine content of various foods. Some examples of these foods and additives are:

- cyclamates
- overly ripe avocados
- monosodium glutamate (MSG)
- preserved meats (e.g., salami, bologna)
- pickled foods (e.g., herring, sauerkraut)
- fermented cheeses (e.g., Blue, Gorgonzola)
- fermented beverages (some beers and wines)
- fermented bean curd products (e.g., soy sauce)

Duration of action

Many MAOIs available in the U.S. inactivate all MAO present in the nerve cell. This means that no MAO is available in the CNS until more is synthesized. For this reason, antidepressant effects are seen for a week or more after the drug is discontinued, or until the nerve cells synthesize adequate amounts of new MAO.

Adverse effects of MAOIs

The most serious risk is the possibility of a hypertensive crisis (see above). A severe headache may signal the onset of a crisis. Other frequent symptoms are:

- increased blood pressure
- *tachycardia* (rapid heartbeat)
- increased body temperature

IMPORTANT: If these symptoms occur, immediate medical attention is required.

These symptoms can indicate a *cardiovascular accident* (stroke or heart attack) which can be fatal. The risk is increased if MAOIs are taken concurrently with common medications such as:

> ## Common MAOIs
> - isocarboxazid/Marplan
> - phenelzine/Nardil
> - selegiline/Eldepryl
>   Emsam(transdermal)
> - tranylcypromine/Parnate
>
> Table 4.4

- any TCA or HCA
- amphetamines or other stimulant drugs
- dextromethorphan (in many cough medicines)
- L-dopa (often prescribed for Parkinson's disease)
- over-the-counter and prescription cold preparations

Ingesting significant quantities of any of these (while on an MAOI) can cause a hypertensive crisis due to increased levels of NE. The usual treatment consists of administering a particular group of antipsychotic drugs (phenothiazines) which block the action of NE.

Other serious adverse effects can occur if MAOIs are combined with other drugs including:

- alcohol
- antihistamines
- barbiturates
- phenothiazine tranquilizers
- narcotics
- insulin

The combination of the drugs listed above and MAOIs can lead to severe *hypotension* (a serious decrease in blood pressure) that also can be fatal. MAOIs are also contraindicated in the presence of liver or kidney disease, cardiovascular disease, asthma, hypertension, and many other diseases.

Due to the difficulties mentioned above, the MAOIs were rarely prescribed. If a patient is taking an MAOI, it is usually because he or she has been on it for many years and the psychiatrist is reluctant to change the medication if it is working.

Transdermal MAOI

There is now available an FDA-approved transdermal (skin patch) MAOI (selegiline/Emsam) that has a much lower risk of serious adverse effects than older, oral MAOIs. At the usual dose selegiline is a relatively selective MAO-B inhibitor; for that reason and because it is transdermal, the dietary restrictions associated with the oral formulations are not necessary.

Patients taking selegiline also report improvement in sexual functioning. The only adverse effect seen was a skin rash at the site of the patch. (This type of rash is common for all transdermal medications and is probably due to the adhesives used.) If this transdermal preparation proves to be safe and effective, MAOIs may become a very useful option for the treatment of depression, particularly for atypical depression or for people who dislike the sexual side effects associated with SSRIs (Bodkin & Amsterdam, 2002).

ATYPICAL ANTIDEPRESSANTS & OTHER TREATMENTS

Below are some antidepressant medications that do not fit neatly into the categories already discussed.

Bupropion

The drug bupropion/Wellbutrin has been found to be useful as an antidepressant medication when used either alone or in combination with SSRIs. The addition of (or switching to) bupropion usually will decrease the sexual dysfunction associated with SSRIs. Patients taking the combination of bupropion and SSRIs reported an increased desire to engage in sexual activity as well as an increased frequency of sexual activity (Clayton, et al., 2004).

Mirtazapine

The drug mirtazapine/Remeron is one of a group of drugs called 5-HT2 serotonin receptor antagonists. Since it is sedating, mirtazapine is frequently used to treat depression when sleep problems and anxiety symptoms are present. There is some evidence that the onset of improvement with mirtazapine is more rapid than with the SSRIs. (Guelfi, et al., 2001).

Discontinuance of antidepressants

With all the antidepressants, after a period of being asymptomatic for six to nine months (after a first episode of depression), the patient, in consultation with the psychiatrist and psychotherapist, may decide to discontinue medication. It is very important that the dose be tapered slowly and the process closely monitored by the prescribing physician.

Atypical Antidepressants
• bupropion/Wellbutrin
• mirtazapine/Remeron
• trazodone/Desyrel
• venlafaxine/Effexor (an SNRI)

Table 4.5

The patient must be cautioned not to stop taking the antidepressant without medical supervision. If the medication is withdrawn too quickly, serious conditions can occur (e.g., delirium, delusions, hallucinations, and on occasion, catatonic states) and a recurrence of the depression is likely (Viguera, et al., 1998).

Olanzapine and other antipsychotic medications

Olanzapine/Zyprexa is an antipsychotic medication rather than an antidepressant that has been shown to be effective as an adjunctive agent for depression (Parker, 2002). The pros and cons for use of the other antipsychotic medications in combination with antidepressants for refractory depression are currently being investigated.

Neuromodulators used to treat depression

Some of the small peptide molecules that exist normally in our bodies are considered neuromodulators. Many hormones fall into this category. The presence and levels of these substances in the nerve cell and the synapse affect behavior by influencing the neuron's response to neurotransmitters.

Thyroid hormone is one example of a neuromodulator. It is well known that the level of thyroid hormone affects mood. *Hypothyroidism* (too little thyroid hormone) is associated with depressed mood, and *hyperthyroidism* (too much thyroid hormone) is associated with anxious states. If the patient's response to antidepressant medication alone is not optimal, psychiatrists may add thyroid hormone or lithium to enhance the antidepressant's effect(s). Other substances known to affect mood which may function as neuromodulators are the *endorphins* (endogenous opiate-like substances), the *corticosteroids,* and hormones such as estrogen, testosterone, and progesterone.

Dehydroepiandrosterone (DHEA)

DHEA has been tested in patients where traditional antidepressant medication either has failed, is not well tolerated, or is not desired by the patient (Binello & Gordon, 2003; Strous, et al., 2003). These studies have shown that DHEA, both alone and in combination with antidepressant medications, may be effective in treating mild to moderate mid-life depressions. These depressions may be due to the decrease in DHEA levels that occurs as we age.

Ketamine, a dissociative anesthetic for depression

Ketamine is a selective and potent N-methyl-d-aspartate (NMDA) receptor antagonist. It is FDA-approved for use as an anesthetic and is used in the treatment of chronic and severe pain (see Chapter 8).

A recent study (Zarate, et al., 2006) showed that a single infusion of ketamine relieved depressive symptoms immediately and robustly and that the relief persisted for several days. This result opens the possibility for development of a new class of antidepressants.

Ketamine is also used recreationally and has potential for abuse. It produces short-lived psychedelic effects and euphoria (see Chapter 9). These psychedelic properties, although experienced by many of the patients in these studies, appear independent of the antidepressant effect. The psychedelic effects occurred within minutes and lasted for less than two hours, whereas the antidepressant effects began as the psychedelic effects subsided and persisted for days (Brown, 2007).

Referenced-EEG (rEEG) to guide medication selection

Even with all of the available choices, about 33% of people with depression do not respond to medication. As of now, there is no method to determine with accuracy which specific medication will work best for any particular patient.

Quantitative EEG (QEEG) or referenced EEG (rEEG) techniques are emerging as possible ways to predict both positive and adverse responses to psychotropic medication (Hoffman, 2006). Hoffman has treated over 200 "hard to treat" patients over the past two years. Using rEEG, he determined that 67% of those tested needed a change in medication or needed a combination of medications that would not have been chosen without the aid of this method. This technique may provide psychiatry with a set of clinically useful biomarkers as a guide for choosing the most appropriate medication for each patient.

ELECTRICAL STIMULATION TREATMENTS

Use of shock to treat mental disorders began centuries ago when hot-cold water immersion and electric-eel therapy were used in the hope of lessening psychiatric symptoms. Chemical and electrical methods were later developed in the forms of insulin shock and electroconvulsive therapy (ECT). Insulin shock was discontinued because it was found to be difficult to control, whereas ECT continues to be refined and is still in use (Avery & Lubrano, 1979; Fink, 2001). Today, more than 100,000 Americans are treated with ECT every year, with ten to twenty times that number world-wide receiving ECT (Fink, 2001).

ECT is the application of an electrical current, usually to one side of the brain, to induce a CNS seizure. ECT is tried when depression is severe or life-threatening, when there are serious contraindications to antidepressant medications, or when medications have already been tried and have not produced improvement. ECT is sometimes used for treating psychotic and schizoaffective disorders when medication has been tried and not been effective. Advantages of ECT include:

- rapidity of response
- no medication side effects
- no risk of suicide due to an overdose
- no interactions with other medications
- possible discontinuance of medication (Avery & Lubrano, 1979; Fink, 2001).

ECT has a negative reputation and is not used as a first-line treatment (although people who have been treated successfully with ECT often request it if they have a relapse). The most frequent adverse effect is the memory-loss that some patients experience after treatment. Some types of memory-loss are difficult to measure with objective tests. Opinions differ as to the seriousness and extent of this effect and how much of the loss is caused by ECT. Impairment of memory after ECT is more severe in the elderly (Avery & Lubrano, 1979; Fink, 2001).

ECT treatment regimen

The ECT treatment regimen usually consists of a series of four to twelve sessions over a period of two to four weeks. ECT is believed to work by inducing a general CNS seizure; drugs are used to suppress motor activity and prevent motor seizures. After the CNS seizure, there is a massive alteration in the availability of transmitter substances. Because there are so many changes in the brain chemistry after ECT, it is difficult to pinpoint the specific cause of relief (Abrams, 2002). Recent studies report neurogenesis and a normalization of metabolism in the hippocampus as a putative cause of the relief (Taylor & Fink, 2006; Wennstrom, et al., 2004).

A full remission or marked improvement is reported in 90% of those treated. Another advantage of ECT is that improvement is rapid, whereas with medication there may be a four-to-twelve week period before the depression lifts completely. If a patient is suicidal, this period can be critical (Abrams, 2002; Avery & Lubrano, 1979; Fink, 2001). Some patients will still require ongoing oral medication after the ECT treatment.

Repetitive transcranial magnetic stimulation (rTMS)

TMS uses a hand-held electrical coil that is placed on the scalp at the location of the left prefrontal cortex. An electrical current is passed through the coil, generating a magnetic pulse that passes through the skull and into the brain. It is believed that the electrical field created leads to a depolarization of neurons in the brain. Although the procedure is similar in some ways to ECT, it is milder and no anesthesia is required. There is some concern that TMS might induce seizures, but so far none have been reported (Kozel & George, 2002). In one study, patients with treatment-resistant depression were treated using TMS. The TMS group had a greater decrease in depressive symptoms than the control group, indicating that TMS has a role in medication-resistant depression (Kozel & George, 2002).

Deep Brain Stimulation (DBS)

DBS is a technique currently being tested for people with treatment-resistant depression. It requires surgical implantation of electrodes into the brain. In a recent study, patients were evaluated for improvement after six months and up to more than four years after implantation. Remission rates were 20% at six months and 40% at last follow-up. The DBS was well-tolerated (Malone, et al., 2009).

Vagus Nerve Stimulation (VNS)

The successful use of VNS as a treatment for epilepsy led to hope that it might also be an effective treatment for depression and bipolar disorder. VNS is a milder version of ECT which requires the implantation of a battery-operated device in the upper left part of the chest. Wires extend from the device and wrap around the vagus nerve at the point where it passes through the neck. The device delivers a mild electrical pulse every five minutes which lasts about 30 seconds. The battery which creates the pulse needs to be replaced every five to ten years requiring an additional surgery.

Patients who were not responsive to antidepressant medications were tested using VNS. After three months of treatment, 30% showed improvement; after a full year of treatment, 45% had improved and 29% had recovered completely (Rush, et al., 2005).

VNS has been found to be as effective as ECT in treating nonpsychotic, depressed patients. Unlike ECT, VNS may increase cognitive performance (Sackheim, et al., 2001). To date, no serious adverse effects from VNS have been observed (Schachter, 2002). VNS was FDA-approved for treatment-resistant depression in 2005.

Direct Relevance to Psychotherapy

There are many different effective ways to intervene when a patient exhibits symptoms of depression. The efficacy of any specific intervention depends on many factors, both situational and personal. When the symptoms are severe, such as when a client is rapidly losing weight or is suicidal, quick relief is essential.

Most experts agree that depression has cognitive, mood, and vegetative components; intervention at any of these levels will affect the depression, and each type of intervention may have different results. Therefore, cognitive therapy, behavior modification, and psychoactive medications may all be appropriate treatments for depression. In fact, any or all of these may be necessary for optimal patient care. It is important to determine whether a referral to a psychiatrist for an evaluation for medication is needed. It appears that medication compliance is greatly improved if there is another mental health professional involved in the treatment regimen.

Sometimes psychotherapists are reluctant to recommend that clients see a psychiatrist for a medication evaluation. Some therapists believe that medication should not be necessary in order to gain relief of symptoms. More often, it is the client who is averse to the idea of taking medication and may have chosen treatment by a psychotherapist, rather than by a psychiatrist, specifically for this reason. It is not unusual for a patient's resistance to taking medication to be one of the most difficult issues in psychotherapy. It is important to take whatever time is necessary to explore these issues as part of psychotherapy.

In addition to their personal biases, both the therapist and the client may be concerned about the costs of a medication evaluation, the necessary lab tests, and the potential ongoing cost of one or more drugs. Also entering into the calculus are the potential adverse effects of taking a medication, and whether the benefits will outweigh any possible harm.

While all of these concerns have some validity, there can be no doubt that the psychotherapist's primary consideration must be to evaluate the facts objectively in order to support the optimal treatment for each client. The symptoms of depression can be severe, and the disease can be life-threatening, so it is essential that the psychotherapist have an open mind and employ objective standards when deciding if a medication evaluation is necessary.

The therapist's direct and thorough assessment of the client's symptoms can be utilized as a diagnostic measure. Referral to a psychiatrist for medication is appropriate if symptoms are severe and have not lessened considerably after three weeks of psychotherapy. Severe symptoms include the presence of suicidal ideation, rapid loss of weight (more than 15 pounds), and an inability to perform normal activities at work, school, or in social settings.

A therapist may believe that taking medication interferes with the therapeutic process and prevents "working through" the underlying cause or causes of the depression. Sometimes a depressed patient who is not on medication will be unable to function in the world, yet when on medication cannot go very deeply into the therapy process. In this situation, the psychotherapist may conclude that the underlying dynamics will not be worked through. Although, on rare occasions this does occur, it is more common that clients who are on medication are both more functional and more capable of doing psychotherapeutic work. In some instances, a client's therapy deepens while on medication due to a decrease in apathy or anxiety, either of which may have been impeding motivation or access to information. A successful course of medication will allow the person to resume a more normal life; this will raise the client's level of self-esteem, which in itself is therapeutic.

When a client is on medication, it is important for a good working relationship to exist between the psychotherapist and the psychiatrist. Since the therapist usually sees the client much more frequently than the psychiatrist does, the therapist will often be the first to notice any significant changes or adverse effects due to medication. It is important for psychotherapists to encourage clients to contact their psychiatrists if symptoms worsen, if adverse side effects appear, or if no improvement is experienced.

All antidepressant medications and electrical stimulation methods can have significant adverse effects and should only be used when the depression is seriously debilitating or the benefit will clearly outweigh any potential harm. Both immediate and long-term consequences must be considered. The determination as to whether any specific medication is appropriate requires the combined efforts of the psychiatrist, who has the expertise in medical assessment and experience with prescribing different drugs, in collaboration with the patient and the psychotherapist.

Often patients who are on antidepressants do not inform the prescribing doctor when they discontinue their medication. The psychotherapist should frequently discuss with patients how they are feeling about their medication, whether they think it is helping, and whether they are still taking it. It is the responsibility of the psychotherapist to inform any client who is considering decreasing or stopping antidepressant medication that this should only be done under medical supervision in order to decrease the likelihood of a recurrence of depressive symptoms and other adverse effects.

Usually, after a patient with a first episode of depression has been asymptomatic for nine months to a year, the psychiatrist, psychotherapist, and patient will consult to determine if it is the right time to try discontinuing the medication. If deemed appropriate, the psychiatrist will work with the patient to develop a schedule for slowly decreasing the dosage. If stopped too rapidly, the depression is likely to recur along with common withdrawal symptoms such as nausea, vomiting, dizziness, chills, sweating, abdominal cramping, diarrhea, insomnia, irritability, and anxiety.

The risk of suicide in depressed patients is greatest four to five months after the most severe symptoms have abated. This is because while in the depths of depression people do not usually have enough energy to commit suicide. If after feeling better for a while a patient's depression returns, or if the depression was not completely resolved, he or she may lose all hope of ever being free of the disease and become suicidal. For this reason, it is advisable to continue medication for at least five months after the depression lifts.

The psychotherapist must always weigh the risks and the benefits of any type of treatment. Some clients are not able to do psychotherapy without medication, and some cannot do psychotherapy with it. You, as the psychotherapist, along with the client and the psychiatrist, will be involved in determining the most appropriate treatment.

References for Chapter 4

Abrams, R. (2002). *Electroconvulsive Therapy.* NY: Oxford Univ. Press.

Arafa, M. & Shamloul, R. (2007). A randomized study examining the effect of 3 SSRIs on premature ejaculation using a validated questionnaire. *Ther. Clin. Risk Manag.*, 3(4), 527–31.

Avery, D. & Lubrano, A. (1979). Depression treated with imipramine and ECT: The DeCarolis study reconsidered. *Am. J. Psychiatry*, 136, 559–562.

Binello, E. & Gordon, C. (2003). Clinical uses and misuses of dehydroepiandrosterone. *Current Opinion Pharmacol.* 3(6), 635-41.

Bodkin, J. & Amsterdam, J. (2002). Transdermal selegiline in major depression: A double-blind, placebo controlled, parallel-group study in out-patients. *Am. J. Psychiatry*, 159, 1869–1875.

Brown, W. (2007). Ketamine and NMDA receptor antagonists for depression. *Psychiatric Times*, 3(2).

Carey, B. (2004), Is Prozac better? Is it even different? Retrieved from http://www.nytimes.com/2004/09/21/health/psychology/21proz.htm

Carey, B. (2005). Antidepressant safety debate may include adult patients. Retrieved from www.nytimes.com/2005/02/18.

Clayton, A., Pradko, J. & Kroft, H. (2002). Prevalence of sexual dysfunction among newer antidepressants. *J. Clin. Psychiatry*, 63, 357–366.

Clayton, A., Warnock, J., Kornstein, S., Pinkerton, R., Sheldon–Keler, A. & McGarvey, E. (2004). A placebo-controlled trial of bupropion SR as an antidote for selective serotonin reuptake inhibitor-induced sexual dysfunction. *J. Clin. Psychiatry*, 65(1), 62–67.

Diler, R., Yolga, A. & Avci, A. (2002). Fluoxetine-induced extrapyramidal symptoms in an adolescent: A case report. *Swiss Med. Wkly.*, 132, 125–126.

Fergusson, D., Doucette, S., Glass, K., Shapiro, S., Healy,D., Hebert, P. & Hutton, B. (2005). Association between suicide attempts and selective serotonin reuptake inhibitors: Systematic review of randomized controlled trials. *BMJ*,

330(7488), 396.

Fink, M. (2001). ECT has much to offer our patients: It should not be ignored. *World J. Biol. Psychiatry*, 2, 1–8.

Fox-Aarons, S., Frances, A. & Mann, J. (1985). Atypical depression: A review of diagnosis and treatment. *Hospital and Community Psychiatry*, 36, 275–282.

Gibbons, R., Brown, C., Hur, K., Marcus, S., Bhaumik, D., Erkens, J., Herings, R., & Mann, J. (2007). Early evidence on the effects of regulators' suicidality warnings on SSRI prescriptions and suicide in children and adolescents. *Am. J. Psychiatry*, 164(9), 1356-363.

Goldstein, D., Lu, Y., Detke, M., Wiltse, C., Mallinckrodt, C. & Demitrack, M. (2004). Duloxetine in the treatment of depression: A double-blind, placebo-controlled comparison with paroxetine. *J. Clin. Psychopharm.* 24(4), 389-399.

Greden, J. (2001). Clinical prevention of recurrent depression. *Review of Psychiatry,* 20(5), 143–170.

Guelfi, J., Ansseau, M., Timmerman, L. & Korsgaard, S. (2001). Mirtazapine versus venlafaxine in hospitalized severely depressed patients with melancholic features. *J. Clin. Psychopharm.*, 20, 531–537.

Hall, W., Mant, A., Mitchell, P., Rendle, V., Hickie, I. & McManus, P. (2003). Association between antidepressant prescribing and suicide in Australia, 1991-2000: Trend analysis. *BMJ*; 1008, 326:

Hoffman, D. (2006). First, do no harm: Predicting a "no medication" response. *J. Neuropsychiatry Clin. Neurosci.*, 18, 256-85, P 17 (Poster presentation).

Kalikow, K. (2008). Psychiatric medications for children: Are we overestimating or underestimating risk and benefit? *Psyc. Times*, Nov., 18-19.

Keller, M., Lavori, P. & Mueller, T. (1992). Time to recovery, chronicity, and levels of psychopathology in major depression. *Arch. Gen. Psychiatry*, 49, 809–816.

Kendler, K. & Prescott, C. (1999). A population-based twin study of lifetime major depression in men and women. *Arch. Gen. Psychiatry*, 56(1), 39–44.

Kozel, F. & George, M. (2002). Meta-analysis of left frontal repetitive transcranial magnetic stimulation (rTMS) to treat depression. *J. Psychiatric Practice*, 8, 270–275.

Lane, R., Baldwin, D., & Preskorn, S. (1995). The SSRIs: Advantages, disadvantages and differences. *J Psychopharmacol.* 9(Suppl.), 163–178.

Lane, R. & Baldwin, D. (1997). Selective serotonin reuptake inhibitor-induced serotonin syndrome. Review. *J. Clinical Psychopharm.*, 17(3), 208–221.

Malone, D., Dougherty, D., Rezai, A., Carpenter, L., Friehs, G., Eskandar, E., Rauch, S., Rasmussen, S., Machado, A. & Kubu C. (2009). Deep Brain Stimulation of the ventral capsule/ventral striatum for treatment-resistant depression. *Biological Psychiatry*, 65(4), 267-75.

Manfredonia, M. (1997). *Psicofarmaci.* {Psychopharmacology} Milan, Italy: il Saggiatore/Flammarion.

Martinez, C., Rietbrock, S., Wise, L., Ashby, D., Chick, J., Moseley, J., Evans, S. & Gunnell, D. (2005). Antidepressant treatment and the risk of fatal and non-fatal self harm in first episode depression: Nested case-control study. *BMJ*, 330(7488), 389.

Mort, J., Aparasu, R. & Baer, R. (2006). Interaction between selective-serotonin reuptake inhibitors and non-steroidal antiinflammatory drugs: Review of the literature. *Pharmacotherapy*, 26, 1307-313.

National Institute of Mental Health (NIMH). Retrieved September 1, 2003 from http://www.surgeongeneral.gov/library/mentalhealth/chapter4/sec3_1.html.

Nemeroff, C., Kalali, A., Keller, M., Charney, D.; Lenderts, S., Cascade, E., Stephenson, H. & Schatzberg, A. (2007). Impact of publicity concerning pediatric suicidality data on physician practice patterns in the United States. *Arch. Gen. Psychiatry,* 64(4), 466-472.

Nurnberg, H., Laurello, J. & Hensley, P. (1999). Sildenafil for sexual dysfunction in women taking antidepressants. *Am. J. Psychiatry*, 156, 1664.

Oquendo, M., Malone, K. & Ellis, S. (1999). Inadequacy of antidepressant treatment for patients with major depression who are at risk for suicidal behavior. *Am. J. Psychiatry*, 156, 190–194.

Parker, G. (2002). Olanzapine augmentation in the treatment of melancholia: The trajectory of improvement in rapid responders. *Int. Clin. Psychopharm.*, 17, 87–89.

Pedersen, L., Henriksen, T., Vestergaard, M., Olsen, J. & Bech, B. (2009). Selective serotonin reuptake inhibitors in pregnancy and congenital malformations: population based cohort study. *BMJ*, 339, b3569.

Perahia, D., Pritchett, Y., Desaiah, D. & Raskin, J. (2006). Efficacy of duloxetine in painful symptoms: An analgesic or anti-depressant effect? *International Clinical Psychopharm.*, 21(6), 311-17.

Roose, S., Glassman, A., Giardina, E., Walsh, B., Woodring, S. & Bigger, J. (1987). Tricyclic antidepressants in depressed patients with cardiac conduction disease. *Arch. Gen. Psychiatry*, 44, 273–275.

Rush, A., Sackeim, H., Marangell, L., George, M., Brannan, S., Davis, S., Lavori, P. & Howland, R. (2005). Effects of 12 months of vagus nerve stimulation in treatment-resistant depression: A naturalistic study. *Biol. Psyc.*, 58, 355-63.

Sackheim, H., Keilp, J. & Rush, S. (2001). The effects of vagus nerve stimulation on cognitive performance in patients with treatment-resistantdepression. *Neuropsyciatry Neuropsychol. Behav. Neurol.*, 14, 53-62.

Schachter, S. (2002). Vagus nerve stimulation: Where are we? *Current Opinion in Neurology*, 15(2), 201–206.

Sheline, Y., Wang, P., Gado, M., Csernansky, J. & Vannier, M. (1996). Hippocampal atrophy in recurrent major depression. *Proc. Natl. Acad. Sci.*, USA 93, 3908–3913.

Strous, R., Mayan, R. & Lapidus, R. & Stryjer R. (2003). DHEA augmentation in the management of negative, depressive, and anxiety symptoms of schizophrenia, *Arch. Gen. Psychiatry*, 60(2), 133-41.

Taylor, M. & Fink, M. (2006). *Melancholia: The Diagnosis, Pathophysiology and Treatment of Depressive Illness.* New York: Cambridge University Press.

Wennstrom, M., Hellsten, J. & Tingstrom, A. (2004). Electroconvulsive seizures induce proliferation of NG2-expressing glial cells in adult rat amygdala. *Biol. Psychiatry*, 55, 464-71.

Zarate, C., Singh, J., Carlson, P., Brutsche, N., Ameli, R., Luckenbaugh, D., Charney, D. & Manji, H. (2006). A randomized trial of an N-methyl-d-aspartate antagonist in treatment-resistant major depression. *Arch. Gen. Psychiatry,* 63, 856-64.

Chapter 5

Treatment of Bipolar Disorder

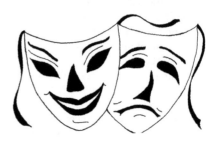

Between two and ten million Americans suffer from bipolar disorder (BD). In adults, BD is typically characterized by a fluctuation between manic and depressed moods, often with no apparent cause for the shift. Most patients find their depressed moods unpleasant and want them to stop, whereas they often want the manic state to continue because it is usually experienced as an invigorating "high." In contrast, friends, relatives, and therapists usually encourage and support all appropriate measures to end a manic state. These "outsiders" have often seen bipolar sufferers getting into severe work, financial, and relationship difficulties due to their manic behaviors. The primary reason many bipolar patients repeatedly cycle in and out of mental hospitals is their unsupervised discontinuance of medication.

The suicide rate for people with untreated bipolar disorder is between ten and 30 times greater than for the general population (Kahn, et al., 1996). Studies show that people with bipolar disorder see an average of three to four doctors and spend more than six years seeking treatment before getting a correct diagnosis (Kaplan, 2007).

There are strong indications of a genetic component in bipolar disorder. If one parent has BD, a child has a 14% risk of developing BD; if both parents have BD, their children's chance of developing the condition is 30% (Kendler & Prescott, 1999; Mota-Castillo & Auvil, 2004).

Childhood bipolar disorder

Diagnosing children with bipolar disorder is very difficult because the symptoms they present are not the same as those seen in adults. Children often seem more agitated and angry, rather than typically manic, and there is a decreased need for sleep.

Between 1994 and 2004 there has been a dramatic increase in the diagnosis of bipolar disorder in children and adolescents, while over that time period the incidence in adults has doubled. The rate in people 19 or younger rose from 25 per 100,000 in 1994 to about 75 per 100,000 in 2004 (Kaplan, 2007). It is not clear if this 300% increase is due to better diagnosis or to over-diagnosis. There is a high degree of comorbidity with attention deficit hyperactivity disorder (ADHD). Children with bipolar disorder often become depressed as adults.

Examples of manic behavior (in adults)

Some typical examples of manic behaviors are:

- restlessness
- argumentativeness
- sexual promiscuity
- reduced need for sleep
- excessive spending
- excessive talking
- excessive gambling
- effusive/expansive mood

It is known that certain stressors, such as substance abuse or lack of sleep, can trigger a manic episode. Mood swings become more frequent during periods without treatment. On average, there are four episodes of mania or depression in the first 10 years of illness. These episodes can last for days, months, or even years. Without treatment, the depression usually lasts about six months. The manic episodes are generally shorter, usually a few months. Some people recover completely between episodes, while others have milder but continuing symptoms of mania or depression.

Cognitive deficits

Some patients with bipolar disorder exhibit cognitive deficits, particularly problems with memory and executive function. Recent brain-imaging findings indicate structural and functional abnormalities in the cortical and limbic networks of the brain in patients with bipolar disorder when compared to healthy controls (Sachs, et al.,

2007). There is some evidence that taking the ACh inhibitors rivastigmine and galantamine may improve cognitive performance in these patients (Hussain, et al., 2003). In adults with BD, current treatment with atypical antipsychotic medication was the best predictor of cognitive impairment (Frangou, et al., 2005). Lithium, anticonvulsants, and antidepressants did not correlate with impaired cognition (Frangou, et al., 2005). Children taking mood-stabilizers (including lithium, anticonvulsants and antipsychotic drugs) performed more poorly than non-medicated children on processing speed and working memory when tested using the WISC-III (Henin, et al., 2009).

Drugs Used to Treat Bipolar Disorder

LITHIUM

The active ingredient in the longest-used medication for the treatment of bipolar disorder is lithium (Li), the third element on the *Periodic Table of Elements*. Lithium can prevent manic episodes, and is somewhat useful (at higher doses) in preventing relapses of depression. It is a better treatment for bipolar illness than for depressive disorders, and is not the first drug of choice for depression.

Sometimes patients with BD who are treated with lithium alone have breakthrough episodes of depression (the depression "breaks through" the preventative treatment). If this occurs, many psychiatrists prescribe lamotrigine (see p. 87) or an antidepressant medication in addition to the lithium (Baldessarini, et al., 2002; Bowden, 1998). When the depression abates, many psychiatrists then taper the patients off the antidepressants, but often will continue the lamotrigine, which is believed to prevent a recurrence of depression (Calabrese, et al.,1999).

Effects of lithium

There is usually a lag period of four to ten days from starting lithium for the antimanic effects to be seen. Behaviors exhibited during a manic episode can be dangerous, and for this reason a patient may be started on an antipsychotic medication to quiet the agitation, while waiting for the antimanic effects of the lithium to begin (Baldessarini, et al., 2002). The antipsychotic medication is then slowly tapered off as the lithium takes effect (generally one to two weeks). After that, antipsychotic medication may not be necessary and is often discontinued (Kahn, et al., 1996).

Lithium has no observable effect on the mood of people who do not have bipolar disorder. It does not cause sedation or euphoria, so it is not likely to be abused. A person taking lithium who is dehydrated (e.g., due to exercising vigorously or perspiring in hot weather) is at a risk of overdose. In dehydrated persons, the concentration of lithium in the blood will increase and the resulting high levels can lead to a comatose state. Similarly, with low-salt diets, a loss of water in the body can cause the blood levels of lithium to increase (Bowden, 1998). To assess for this, and to determine therapeutic dose, the blood levels of patients on lithium must be carefully monitored.

Blood levels of lithium can now be determined in minutes with a test performed in the doctor's office. The test uses just a few drops of blood obtained from a finger-stick (Kaplan, 2005). This new test eliminates the difficulty and expense of obtaining accurate blood levels, which had been one of the major obstacles to using lithium.

Between 70% to 90% of bipolar disorder sufferers respond well to lithium, although it can take months to find the correct dose (Baldessarini, et al., 2002). The lag in response time is one reason why the psychotherapist and the prescribing psychiatrist need to be in communication with each other. Bipolar patients are often not the best judges of whether their medication is helping during this period. The therapist will need to provide the psychiatrist with objective feedback as to how the patient seems to be responding to the medication and whether any adverse effects are observed.

It is not yet clear exactly how lithium works to decrease the symptoms of BD, but it is believed to promote neuronal growth. Lithium also may protect neurons from cell death and increase the volume of gray matter in the limbic system (Bearden, et al., 2007).

Adverse effects of lithium

Taking lithium can cause many adverse effects, including:

- **Kidney damage:** When taken over long periods, lithium may cause serious kidney damage. For this reason, it is important that kidney functioning be carefully monitored by a medical doctor, preferably a psychiatrist. If kidney damage occurs, the patient must be taken off lithium and switched to a different drug that will control the manic behavior and not damage the kidneys (Bowden, 1998, Dunn, et al., 1998, Pope, et al., 1991).

- **Thyroid functioning:** To rule out thyroid problems as an underlying cause of depressive or manic symptoms, many psychiatrists require a thyroid panel before starting any medication. Lithium may inhibit thyroid functioning. When hypothyroidism develops in response to lithium, it is usually remedied by prescribing thyroid hormone. If lithium is taken long-term, hypothyroidism will occur in approximately 15% of patients (Bowden, 1998). Irregularities in thyroid functioning can lead to either hyperactive or depressive symptoms. These symptoms can be similar to depression or mania. Lab tests for thyroid levels are usually required to differentiate between medication effects and an underlying thyroid condition. Thyroid functioning will return to normal when lithium is discontinued (Bowden, 1998).

- **Altered glucose metabolism:** Lithium alters glucose tolerance, the complex metabolic process that regulates the absorption of glucose into blood and tissues via the insulin mechanism. Even patients who are not diabetic can develop a condition of mild diabetes while taking lithium. A person known to be diabetic before starting lithium requires careful monitoring to determine whether an adjustment in the usual dose of insulin is needed. The prescribing psychiatrist must carefully monitor these medical conditions and adjust the levels of lithium and/or insulin as is appropriate (Bowden, 1998).

ANTICONVULSANT MEDICATIONS FOR BIPOLAR DISORDER

Although most are not FDA-approved as a maintenance treatment for bipolar disorder, many anticonvulsant drugs are used to control manic symptoms. Anticonvulsant medications are often used as an alternative to lithium for the treatment of bipolar disorder for patients who do not respond to lithium, for patients who are allergic to lithium, or for those who cannot tolerate lithium's adverse effects. About 30% of people with bipolar disorder fall into one of these categories (Pope, et al., 1991).

Anticonvulsant or antipsychotic drugs, in combination with lithium, are also used for patients whose manic symptoms do not abate with lithium alone. These drugs are very useful in the treatment of acute manic states because they take effect more quickly than lithium (Dunn, et al., 1998). Anticonvulsants are less effective than lithium in preventing depressive episodes (Baldessarini, et al., 2002).

Divalproex is FDA-approved for its primary use as an antiseizure medication and also for the treatment of acute manic episodes (Pope, et al., 1991).

Lamotrigine/Lamictal is an anticonvulsant drug that is now FDA-approved for the maintenance treatment of bipolar disorder (see p. 87).

Adverse effects of anticonvulsant drugs

One danger in the use of anticonvulsant medications is that they can have the paradoxical effect of inducing a seizure if the dose is raised too quickly. Taking anticonvulsant drugs may also worsen any cardiac conduction disease already present (although these drugs are less cardiotoxic than TCAs and HCAs) (Dunn, et al., 1998). Most anticonvulsants are also known to cause birth defects when taken during pregnancy.

The anticonvulsant drugs (except for lamotrigine) are not useful for the treatment of the depressive aspect of bipolar disorder.

Teratogenic effects (birth defects)

There is evidence that all of the drugs for BD can cause fetal malformations if taken during pregnancy (Viguera, et al., 2002). Women taking these medications need to be informed about possible teratogenic effects. A recent study done in Finland of pregnant women on anticonvulsant medication found major malformations (neural tube defects, oral clefts, cardiovascular and visceral malformations) at a rate 14 times greater than in the rest of the Finnish population. Drugs taken by the women included divalproex, carbamazepine, and oxcarbazepine. Women with epilepsy who were not taking antiseizure medication had a rate of fetal malformations similar to the rates seen in women who do not have epilepsy (Kaaja, 2003).

Effects on male reproductive function

Carbamazepine, oxcarbazepine and divalproex have been found to be associated with sperm abnormalities. Men treated with divalproex had both abnormal sperm and reduced testicular size (Isojarvi, et al., 2004).

Carbamazepine, adverse effects

Carbamazepine/Tegretol can cause hematological disturbances such as *aplastic anemia* (a decrease in all types of blood cells) and *agranulocytosis* (a decrease in the type of white blood cells called granulocytes). Each of these blood disorders is seen in about one in every 20,000 patients treated. Aplastic anemia and agranulocytosis occur with about equal frequency. Both conditions can be fatal.

During the first few weeks of use, carbamazepine can cause *hepatitis* (inflammation of the liver), which can be fatal if it is not detected early and the drug discontinued. It can also cause:

- nausea
- vomiting
- diarrhea
- gastric distress
- anorexia
- constipation

Gabapentin, adverse effects

Since gabapentin/Neurontin is sedating, it is often chosen for patients who are more agitated or have ongoing sleep difficulties.

Although prescribed to treat bipolar disorder, gabapentin is not FDA-approved for this use. Taking gabapentin can cause:

- sleepiness
- dizziness
- fatigue
- nausea
- vomiting
- unsteadiness

Valproate (divalproex sodium, valproic acid), adverse effects

The side effects of valproate/Depakene/Depakote are similar to those of other anticonvulsants (see above). Tolerance to these effects usually develops after a few weeks. Blood disorders that result in prolongation of bleeding time also have been observed. There are other serious, adverse effects involving the pancreas and liver. Rare but serious cases of pancreatitis (inflammation of the pancreas), occasionally resulting in death, have been reported (Pope, et al., 1991).

Taking divalproex can also cause:

- vomiting
- weight gain
- nausea
- hair loss
- sedation
- tremor

An important study (Goodwin, et al., 2003) compared the medical records of 20,638 patients with bipolar disorder who were taking either lithium or divalproex. The researchers found that the patients taking divalproex were 2.7 times more likely to commit suicide than those taking lithium. This study indicates that lithium should be considered the first drug of choice for the treatment of bipolar disorder.

Since the 2003 publication of Goodwin's study, the best way to treat bipolar disorder has been actively debated. The issue is not yet resolved. It may turn out that there is no "best way" and that every patient should be evaluated individually with respect to presenting symptoms and relevant medical risks and benefits.

NEWER ANTICONVULSANT DRUGS

Lamotrigine

Lamotrigine/Lamictal, an antiseizure drug, is FDA-approved for maintenance therapy in bipolar disorder and for the prevention of the

Anticonvulsant Medications

- carbamazepine/Carbatrol, Tegretol
- gabapentin/Neurontin
- lamotrigine/Lamictal
- topiramate/Topamax
- valproate/Depakene, Depakote

Table 5.1

recurrent depressive episodes that may occur with this disorder. It is more effective than lithium in preventing recurrence of depressive episodes (Bowden, et al., 2003). The main adverse effect of this drug is that it can cause a serious allergic reaction known as Stevens-Johnson Syndrome (SJS), a toxic epidermal necrosis. SJS occurs most frequently when the dose is increased too rapidly. It occurs in one in 1,000 adults and in as many as 1% to 2% of children. The syndrome is usually alleviated by decreasing the dose. Frequently, the medication can be reinstated and the dose increased more slowly without the symptoms returning.

Topiramate

Yet another antiseizure drug, topiramate/Topamax, is now being used as a mood stabilizer to treat bipolar disorder. Topiramate is not FDA-approved for the treatment of bipolar disorder. Like most other antiseizure drugs, it is useful in controlling manic episodes and has the advantage of taking effect more quickly than lithium (Dunn, et al., 1998).

The main advantage to this drug is that it does not cause the weight gain experienced with other drugs for bipolar disorder and may in fact induce weight loss. If a person is started on this drug there will not be the issue of obesity and metabolic syndrome (side effects that are present with other mood stabilizing medications). According to the manufacturer, weight loss has occurred in up to 90% of patients taking topiramate. This effect may be dose-related. Up to 7% of weight has been lost in higher dose ranges (600 to 1000mg/day). (This is equivalent to a loss of up to 21 lbs. for a 300 pound person.) Patients may be very sedated at these higher doses. Depending on the individual, the weight loss may be experienced as positive or negative, and may or may not be beneficial to health. There is evidence that topiramate is also effective in treating and preventing cluster headaches (Lainez, et al., 2003).

The most common adverse effects of topiramate are:

- speech or language problems
- dizziness or balance problems
- feeling sluggish, sedated, confused
- feelings of being unusually tired or weak
- irregular eye movements and double-vision
- oligohidrosis (excessive sweating and hyperthermia), especially in pediatric patients (Dunn, et al., 1998)
- memory difficulties • nervousness • tremor

ANTIPSYCHOTIC MEDICATIONS FOR BIPOLAR DISORDER

For many years, various antipsychotic medications have been used without FDA approval to treat mania. These drugs have the advantage of controlling manic symptoms more rapidly than lithium. Sedation is usually immediate, and general improvement can be seen one week after the start of medication.

Recently, some antipsychotic medications have received FDA-approval for treatment of bipolar disorder. The first in this group to be approved by the FDA for acute mania and bipolar maintenance was olanzapine/Zyprexa. Since then, risperidone and quetiapine have received approval for the treatment of acute mania. Aripiprazole is now approved for both acute and maintenance treatment of the manic and mixed episodes associated with Bipolar I disorder, with or without psychotic features (both for adults and for pediatric patients 10 to 17 years of age). Ziprasidone is now approved for the acute manic or mixed episodes associated with bipolar disorder, with or without psychotic features. Olanzapine and fluoxetine have been combined in a compound called Symbyax, which has been approved for the treatment of bipolar depression. These drugs may also be useful for people who cannot tolerate either lithium or the anticonvulsants.

Treatment of bipolar depression

The use of antidepressant medications in maintenence therapy for BD remains controversial. A review of recent research by Ghaemi & Filkowski (2006) concluded that antidepressants are effective in only about 15-20% of patients with BD and that their use is likely to lead to a worsened course of illness in those with rapid-cycling BD.

Obesity in bipolar disorder

People with BD tend to be more overweight than the general population and are more likely to have abdominal obesity. This is believed to be due to both binge-eating by people with bipolar disorder and side effects of the medications used to treat BD.

Lithium is associated with a weight gain that occurs within the first two years of treatment, often more than 10 lbs. Divalproex is associated with a weight gain of more than 44 lbs. (depending on length of treatment). Weight gain with a combination of lithium and divalproex is additive. Divalproex and lithium are each associated with more weight gain than carbamazepine (Elmslie, et al., 2000, Nemeroff, 2003).

Gabapentin is associated with an increase of more than 10 percent of body weight in more than 25% of patients. Weight gain was not an issue with lamotrigine and weight loss was common with topiramate. Topiramate seems to decrease the frequency of binge-eating (Kotwal, et al., 2003, McElroy, et al., 2003).

Emerging therapies

The pharmacological treatment of bipolar disorder is complex, and there are few FDA-approved drugs for BD that adequately control both the manic and depressive phases of the disorder. Many of the drugs currently used for BD are FDA-approved for other indications and are being used "off-label" for BD. This does not mean that they are not good choices to control BD symptoms. It does usually mean that there have not been large, placebo-controlled studies using these drugs specifically to treat BD or that the studies that have been done have may have been financed by the company that manufactures the drug.

There are several drugs currently under study in independent clinical trials, which may prove to be safe and effective for BD. Two of these are discussed below.

Riluzole

Riluzole is FDA-approved under the brand name Rilutek for the treatment of *amyotrophic lateral sclerosis* (ALS), also known as Lou Gehrig's disease. Riluzole is being evaluated for use in treating depressive symptoms in patients with BD. This study is based on research (Du, et al., 2007) that found that riluzole may have a mechanism of action similar to lamotrigine, which is already known to be effective in reducing depressive symptoms in BD.

Tamoxifen

A research study (Yildiz, et al., 2008) investigated the effectiveness of using tamoxifen to treat mania in patients with BD. This was a placebo-controlled study with seriously ill patients. After three weeks, mania decreased significantly in the subjects receiving the tamoxifen and increased in the subjects receiving the placebo. Tamoxifen may prove to be a well-tolerated, inexpensive treatment for BD and may have fewer and more benign adverse effects than other drugs currently available.

Direct Relevance to Psychotherapy

Most therapists agree that it is not possible to do psychotherapy with a client who is in a manic state. People in a manic state usually do not perceive problems with their behavior or feelings and therefore seldom see any need for medication or treatment. Paranoid delusions are often present, making it difficult to create and maintain a therapeutic alliance. Before effective psychotherapy can take place, the manic episode must be terminated.

There is evidence that cognitive therapy (CT), when used as an adjunct to medication, significantly reduces the rate of relapse in

Bipolar I patients. In one study, therapists taught their clients how to monitor themselves for prodromal symptoms of relapse, to maintain regular schedules, and to moderate their attempts to compensate for the time they lost from work when feeling ill. Patients receiving CT had better medication compliance, better social functioning, fewer manic swings, and fewer hospitalizations than those in the control group (Lam, 2003).

All antimanic drugs have adverse effects that can be serious and sometimes fatal. It is very likely that psychotherapists, because they often have more frequent contact with clients than psychiatrists, will be the first to recognize a serious adverse effect due to medication. For this reason, a collaborative relationship between the therapist and the prescribing psychiatrist is crucial when treating patients with bipolar disorder.

References for Chapter 5

Baldessarini, R., Tondo, L., Hennen, J. & Viguera, A. (2002). Is lithium still worth using? An update of selected recent research. *Harvard Rev. Psychiatry*, 10, 59–75.

Bowden, C. (1998). Key treatment studies of lithium in manic-depressive illness: Efficacy and side effects. *J. Clin. Psychiatry*, 59(Suppl. 6), 13–20.

Bearden, C., Thompson, P., Dalwani, M., Hayashi, K., Lee, A., Nicoletti, M., Trakhtenbroit, M., Glahn, D., Brambilla, P., Sassi, R., Mallinger, A., Frank, E., Kupfer, D. & Soares, J. (2007). Greater cortical gray matter density in lithium-treated patients with bipolar disorder. *Biol Psychiatry*, 62:7.

Bowden, C., Calabrese, J., Sachs, G.,Yatham, L., Asghar, S., Hompland, M., Montgomery, P., Earl, N., Smoot, T. & DeVeaugh-Geiss, J. (2003). A placebo-controlled 18 month trial of lamotrigine and lithium maintenence treatment in recently manic or hypomanic patients with bipolar I disorder. *Arch. Gen. Psychiatry*, 60, 392-400.

Calabrese, J., Bowden, C., Sachs, G., Ascher, J., Monaghan, E., Rudd, G. Lamictal 602 Study Group. (1999). A double-blind placebo-controlled study of lamotrigine monotherapy in outpatients with bipolar I depression. *J. Clin. Psychiatry*, 60(2), 79-88.

Du, J., Suzuki K., Wei, Y., Wang, Y., Blumenthal, R., Chen, Z., Falke, C., Zarate, C. Jr. & Manji, H. (2007). The anticonvulsants lamotrigine, riluzole, and valproate differentially regulate AMPA receptor membrane localization: Relationship to clinical effects in mood disorders. *Neuropsychopharm.*, 32, 793-802.

Dunn, R., Frye, M., Kimbrell, T., Denicoff, K. Leverich, G.& Post, R. (1998). The efficacy and use of anticonvulsants in mood disorders. *Clinical Neuropharm.*,

21, 215–235.

Elmslie, J., Silverstone, J., Mann, J., Williams, S. & Romans, S. (2000). Prevalence of overweight and obesity in bipolar patients. *J. Clin. Psyc.*,61(3), 179-84.

Frangou, S., Donaldson, S., Hadjulis, M., Landau, S. & Goldstein, L. (2005). The Maudsley Bipolar Disorder Project: Executive dysfunction in bipolar disorder I and its clinical correlates. *Biol. Psychiatry*, 58, 859-64.

Ghaemi, S. & Sachs, G. (1997). Long term risperidone treatment in bipolar disorder: 6-month follow up. *Int. Clin. Psychopharmacol.*, 12, 333–338.

Ghaemi, S. & Filkowski, M. (2006). Antidepressants and bipolar disorder: What do recent studies tell us? *Psyc. Times*, XXIII(6), 66-70.

Goodwin, K., Fireman, B., Simon, G., Hunkeler, E., Lee, J. & Revicki, D. (2003). Suicide risk in bipolar disorder during treatment with lithium and divalproex. *JAMA*, 290(11), 1467–1473.

Guille, C., Sachs, G. & Ghaemi, S. (2000). A naturalistic comparison of clozapine, risperidone, and olanzapine in the treatment of bipolar disorder. *J. Clin. Psychiatry*, 61, 638–642.

Henin, A., Mick, E., Biederman, J., Fried, R., Hirshfeld-Becker, D., Micco, J., Miller, K., Rycyna, C. & Wozniak, J. (2009). Is psychopharmacologic treatment associated with neuropsychological deficits in bipolar youth? *J. Clin. Psychiatry*, 70(8), 1178-85.

Hussain, M., Chaudry, Z. & Hussain, S. (2003). Rivastigmine tartrate and galantamine in neurocognitive deficits in bipolar mood disorder. *156th Annual Meeting of the American Psychiatric Association*, May, 2003, San Francisco.

Isojarvi, J., Lofgren, E., Juntunen, K., Pakarinen, A., Paivansalo, M., Rautakorpi, I. & Tuomivaara, L. (2004). Effect of epilepsy and antiepileptic drugs on male reproductive health. *Neurology*, 62, 247–253.

Kaaja, E (2003). Fetal malformations. *Neurology*, 60, 575–579.

Kahn, D., Ross, R., Rush, A. & Panico, S. (1996). Expert consensus guidelines for bipolar disorder: A guide for patients and families. *J. Clin. Psychiatry*, 57(Suppl. 12A), 81–88.

Kaplan, A. (2005). FDA-approved office lithium test expected to enhance clinical care. *Psyc. Times*, XXII(9), 1, 6-7.

Kaplan, A. (2007). Increase in bipolar diagnosis in youth prompts debates and call for research. *Psyc. Times*, XXIV(14), 1, 6-8.

Kendler, K. & Prescott, C. (1999). A population-based twin study of lifetime major depression in men and women. *Arch. Gen. Psychiatry*, 56(1), 39–44.

Kotwal, R., Guerdjikova, A., McElroy, S. & Keck, P. (2006). Lithium augmentation of topiramate for bipolar disorder with comorbid binge eating disorder and obesity. *Human Psychopharmacology: Clinical and Experimental*, 21(7), 425–431.

Lainez, M., Pascual, J., Pascual, A., Santonja, J., Ponz, A. & Salvador, A. (2003). Topiramate in the prophylactic treatment of cluster headache. *Headache*, 43, 784–789.

Lam, D. (2003). Cognitive therapy for relapse prevention for bipolar disorder. *Arch. Gen. Psych.*, 60, 145–152.

McElroy, S., Arnold, L., Shapira, N., Keck, P., Jr., Rosenthal, N., Rezaul Karim, M., Kamin, M. & Hudson, J. (2003). Topiramate in the treatment of binge eating disorder associated with obesity: A randomized, placebo-controlled trial. *Am. J. Psychiatry,* 160, 255-61.

Mota-Castillo, M. & Auvil, E. (2004). Bipolar disorder and genetics: Beyond question, *Psyc. Times,* (June), 21-22.

Nemeroff, C. (2003). Safety of available agents used to treat bipolar disorder: Focus on weight gain. *J. Clin. Psyc.,* 64(5), 532-39.

Periodic Table of the Elements. Retrieved October 12, 2003, from http://www.webelements.com/

Pope, H. Jr., Mc Elroy, S. Keck, P. & Hudson, J. (1991). Valproate in the treatment of acute mania: A placebo controlled study. *Arch. Gen. Psychiatry,* 48, 62–68.

Sachs, G., Schaffer, M. & Winklbaur, B. (2007). Cognitive deficits in bipolar disorder. *Neuropsychiatr.,* 21(2),93-101.

Viguera, A., Cohen, L., Baldessarini, R. & Nonacs, R. (2002). Managing bipolar disorder during pregnancy: Weighing the risks and benefits. *Can. J. Psychiatry,* 47, 426–436.

Yildiz, A., Guleryuz, S., Ankerst, D., Öngür, D. & Renshaw, P. (2008). Protein kinase C inhibition in the treatment of mania: A double-blind, placebo-controlled trial of tamoxifen. *Arch.Gen. Psychiatry,* 65(3), 255-63.

Chapter 6

CNS Stimulants: Use & Abuse

I love coffee, I love tea
I love the java jive and it loves me
Coffee and tea and the jivin' and me
A cup, a cup, a cup, a cup, a cup!
"*Java Jive*," 1940

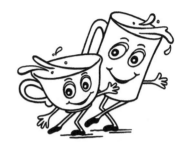

The class of drugs designated as central nervous system (CNS) stimulants includes the two most frequently-used drugs on the planet, caffeine and nicotine. This chapter also includes all the amphetamines, cocaine, modafinil/Provigil, and the drugs approved to treat attention deficit hyperactivity disorder (ADHD) in children and adults, namely atomoxetine/Strattera, methylphenidate/Ritalin/Concerta/Daytrana, and the prodrug lisdexamfetamine/Vyvanse.

General Effects of Stimulants

All stimulant drugs cause an increase in general behavioral activity. When taken short-term (one or two weeks), stimulant drugs cause states of euphoria, optimism, and general feelings of well-being. Initial feelings of anorexia are frequent, a quality that leads to their use/abuse in weight loss products. Insomnia is also frequent. These responses indicate that the part of the brain which controls these functions, the hypothalamus, is strongly affected by these drugs and that the dopamine transmitter system is primarily involved in many of these effects. Other effects are:

- decreased feelings of depression
- increased thoughts and associations
- increased talkativeness • increased blood pressure
- anxiety • irritability • decreased fatigue

Tolerance to stimulants

Tolerance to the mood-elevating and appetite-suppressing effects develops after about two weeks of daily use. Little tolerance develops to the behavioral-arousal effect, which is what makes these drugs useful in the long-term treatment of narcolepsy (Stahl, 1999).

Abuse of Stimulants & Treatments for Withdrawal

A person who is addicted to stimulants, or who has had a long period of continuous use, will experience withdrawal symptoms if the drug is stopped abruptly. Symptoms of withdrawal from amphetamines and cocaine are very similar, mainly feelings of depression, fatigue, apathy, and general sluggishness, the opposite of the effects seen under the influence of these drugs. These symptoms, though not physically dangerous, can be very uncomfortable (Chiang & Goldfrank, 1990).

If a depressed person has been using stimulants on a long-term basis, has become dependent, or is abusing these drugs and increasing the dosage, then a severe depression may occur when the drug is withdrawn (Chiang & Goldfrank, 1990). If the depression caused by withdrawal does not abate after a week or two, evaluation by a psychiatrist for antidepressant medication is appropriate.

AMPHETAMINES

Amphetamine, dextroamphetamine, and methamphetamine (collectively referred to as "amphetamines") all have very similar properties and effects. The first amphetamine was synthesized in 1887, but it was not until the 1920s that it was investigated as a treatment for a wide variety of ills such as depression and nasal decongestion. In the 1930s, an inhaler, "Benzedrine" (mixed amphetamine sulfate), was sold over-the-counter and marketed for the treatment of asthma, hay fever, and the common cold. Methamphetamine (MA), discovered in 1919, is a crystalline powder that is easy to make (this is the "speed," "crank," or "meth" often made in illegal drug labs). It can be smoked, snorted, injected when dissolved in water, or taken in pill form. During World War II, amphetamines were sometimes used to push soldiers to their limits, and even today "go pills" are used by U.S. military pilots to keep them awake when on long missions. Dextroamphetamine/Dexedrine and methamphetamine/Desoxyn were widely available in the 1950s and were popular with truck drivers and college students for staying awake, used by athletes to enhance performance, and taken and by millions as an appetite suppressant (Methamphetamine information, 2003).

Researchers may have discovered a reason why men have higher rates of addiction than women; male brains release up to three times more dopamine than female brains in response to amphetamine use. The men released between 50% and 200% more than the average females in the study. This may help explain the sex disparity in addictions (Munro, et al., 2006).

Methamphetamine addiction does destroy brain cells

In one study, high resolution MRI scans of methamphetamine addicts showed tissue destruction, particularly in gray matter. Losses were seen in the limbic region and the hippocampus. The study looked at 22 subjects who had used an average of four grams of methamphetamine per week for ten years, mostly by smoking it (Thompson, et al., 2004).

Psychological effects of methamphetamine use

Long-term users of methamphetamine frequently develop a variety of psychotic symptoms. These can be auditory hallucinations, paranoia, delusions, and formication (the illusion that insects are crawling on or under the skin) (Rawson & Ling, 2007).

Treatment of methamphetamine dependence

There are no FDA-approved drugs for methamphetamine dependence or withdrawal. A few currently in clinical trials are:

- Bupropion/Wellbutrin was shown to be somewhat helpful in increasing the number of drug-free weeks for low to moderate methamphetamine users (Elkashef, et al., 2008).

- Mirtazapine/Remeron has shown promise for the treatment of withdrawal symptoms (McGregor, et al., 2005).

- Gamma-vinyl-GABA (GVG) (see p. 99) has shown some effectiveness keeping methamphetamine users drug free for at least four weeks. (Brodie, et al., 2005).

- Modafinil/Provigil was reported to decrease the severity of withdrawal symptoms. Subjects reported deeper sleep, fewer nightmares, and less sleepiness during the day (McGregor, et al., 2005).

All of these drugs may eventually prove to be helpful. However, larger, placebo-controlled trials are necessary to confirm their effectiveness.

COCAINE

Evidence suggests that the coca plant, *Erythroxylum coca,* was domesticated in South America around 1500 BCE. To this day, coca is an important part of many cultures in the Andes, where it is used in social rituals and its leaves are chewed to provide stimulation and relief from hunger. The plant's active ingredient, cocaine, was isolated by chemists in 1860. In the latter half of the 19th century, cocaine was considered to be an elixir, and was included in many patent medicines.

Coca-Cola®, which takes its name from the coca plant, included cocaine as an ingredient when it was introduced in 1885, which helped to make Coke® the world's most popular soft drink. The cocaine was removed in 1903 as its dangers began to be recognized (Krol, 2003).

Cocaine ("coke," "crack") is a potent CNS stimulant which is biochemically similar to the amphetamines and produces similar (although shorter-lasting) mood-elevating effects. The behavioral effects of cocaine are also similar to those of the amphetamines. Various formulations of cocaine (Novocaine, Lidocaine, Carbocaine, etc.) have been used as local anesthetics for many years.

Cocaine can be lethal, particularly if taken by injection. Fatality can result from heart failure, respiratory depression, stroke, or seizures (Chiang, & Goldfrank, 1990). People have been known to die the first time they try cocaine, usually from previously unknown heart defects.

Brompton's cocktail

Brompton's cocktail is a medicinal concoction of cocaine, methadone, and alcohol. It is used with terminally-ill patients to alleviate extreme pain. The cocaine counteracts the sedation caused by the methadone. Brompton's cocktail is not used more generally because it has the potential to be highly addictive due to the rapid onset of stimulant and euphoric effects (McGiverny & Crooks, 1984).

Psychotic symptoms in cocaine users

In terms of psychological effects, cocaine use can produce a psychosis that is indistinguishable from the psychosis seen with paranoid schizophrenia. The best way to distinguish between these is either to run a blood test for cocaine, or wait until the drug should have worn off and see if the psychotic symptoms abate.

A treatment dilemma may occur if a cocaine user is also having psychotic symptoms and needs to be treated with an antipsychotic drug. Administration of antipsychotic drugs leads to increased cravings for cocaine. This is probably due to the blocking of dopamine receptors caused by the antipsychotic medication. The cravings may lead to an increase in cocaine use, which then may lead to a worsening of psychotic symptoms (Chiang & Goldfrank, 1990).

TREATMENTS FOR COCAINE DEPENDENCE

Currently there are no FDA approved medications for treatment of cocaine dependence. Some drugs that are currently undergoing clinical trials are discussed below. All of the proposed mechanisms of action for these drugs are very hypothetical.

Gamma-vinyl-GABA (GVG)

GVG is an antiepileptic drug which has been shown to reduce cocaine cravings. It is believed to work by enhancing GABA transmission in the CNS. The usual side effects are sleepiness and fatigue. It is not approved for use in the U.S. but it is available in Canada and other countries (Gerasimov, et al., 2000; Peng, et al., 2008).

Disulfiram

Disulfiram/Antabuse has been evaluated as a treatment for individuals with comorbid alcohol and cocaine abuse. Disulfiram-treated subjects decreased the quantity and frequency of their cocaine use significantly more than those treated with placebo (Petrakis, et al., 2000). The specific mechanism for this effect is not yet clear (Kampman, 2005).

Gabapentin

Gabapentin/Neurontin is an antiepileptic drug which appears to be safe and effective in reducing cocaine usage. Gabapentin is hypothesized to reduce cocaine use by its action on GABA and dopamine pathways in the brain (Raby & Coomaraswamy, 2004).

Topiramate

Topiramate/Topamax may help with relapse prevention due to its effects on both GABA and glutamate neurotransmission. Topiramate increases cerebral levels and facilitates neurotransmission of GABA (Kuzniecky, et al., 1998, Petroff, et al., 1999). Topiramate also inhibits glutamate neurotransmission (Gibbs, et al., 2000).

Modafinil

One study compared the use of cognitive-behavioral therapy to a combination of cognitive-behavioral therapy and modafinil/Provigil with subjects in recovery from cocaine use. Those subjects receiving both modafinil and CBT were more likely to remain cocaine-free than those receiving CBT alone (Dackis, et al., 2003). Modafinil may work by ameliorating glutamate depletion seen in chronic cocaine users (Dackis, et al., 2005).

Cocaine vaccine

A vaccine is being tested that induces the formation of antico-caine antibodies. The antibodies combine with cocaine to form a large molecular complex which has difficulty crossing the blood-brain barrier; this leads to a decrease in the amount of cocaine that penetrates the brain. The impact on the pleasure centers is greatly diminished if only a small amount of cocaine gets into the brain. In animal models, addiction was extinguished using these methods. The anticocaine antibodies remain in the blood and are effective for six months to one year, after which time booster shots might be required.

One danger with this treatment is that very large doses of cocaine might be able to overcome the antibodies which could lead to a lethal overdose. If effective, it is hoped that the vaccine will be a valuable adjunct to psychotherapy for cocaine users who want to overcome their addiction (Orson, et al., 2008; Sussman, 1997).

Relapse Prevention therapy/Harm-Reduction model

Relapse Prevention therapy (RP) (also known as the Harm-Reduction model) is one of the few scientifically validated psychosocial treatments for substance abuse that has been proven useful for treatment of cocaine abuse. No other type of currently available treatment is without major difficulties or side effects. RP techniques help people recognize high-risk situations, rehearse ways to deal with them, self-monitor substance use, and learn to deal with cravings by understanding and discussing them.

With this type of therapy, lapses in behavior are regarded as learning tools (i.e., ways to understand what happened) as well as opportunities to renew the commitment to sobriety. RP does not result in greater total abstinence rates than other treatments, but relapses are shorter. RP may be better in the long term for maintaining a lower relapse rate (Carpenter, 2001; Foxhall, 2001).

CAFFEINE

Coffee and tea are the most common sources of caffeine. Tea is made from the leaves of the *Camellia sinensis* plant and is believed to have been in use in China since about 2700 BCE. The legend is that a servant of the emperor was boiling water when the leaf of an overhead tree dropped into the water, and the emperor decided to taste it (Golender & Bouquet, 2003). He must have liked it.

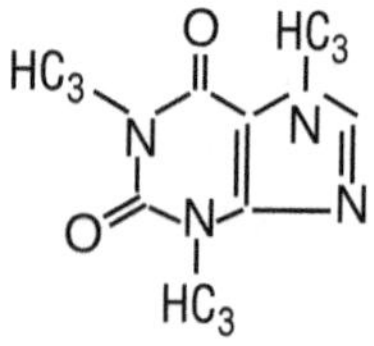

$(C_8H_{10}N_4O_2)$
caffeine

Fig. 6.1

Coffee is made from the berries of species of the genus *Coffea*, in particular *Coffea arabica* and *Coffea canephora*. One legend says that its stimulant property was discovered by a shepherd who observed his flock becoming hyperactive after eating the bright red berries. Coffee has been consumed as a beverage in Middle Eastern cultures since about 1100 CE. When it was introduced to Europe in about 1600, many considered it the "devil's drink" because it was popular in non-Christian societies. Then the pope tried it, and he liked it so much he "baptized" it, thereby removing its stigma (The coffee plant, 2003).

Caffeine is the most widely-used psychoactive substance. Eighty-nine percent of adults in the U.S. use a caffeinated beverage daily. The average user consumes approximately 1,000 cups per year (about three cups per day). Most people do not think of it as a drug, but caffeine is a powerful stimulant. Although its use is legal, overdosing on caffeine, though it might be difficult (more than 5 to 10 grams at one time), can be fatal. Caffeine is quite addicting; tolerance and a tendency to increase intake are common, and withdrawal symptoms will occur if consumption is stopped (Hughes, et al., 1991).

Because caffeine makes people feel better in general, it is often included as an ingredient in analgesics (e.g., Anacin, Excedrin) as well as in many cold preparations. Caffeine intake can be estimated using Table 6.1 (amounts are approximate, and the caffeine content will vary depending on the product and the method of preparation).

Effects of caffeine

Caffeine causes an increase in cellular activity in the CNS and behavioral and emotional responses that are similar to, but milder than, the amphetamines and cocaine. After consuming caffeine, people report thinking more clearly, having more energy, and having faster reaction times (Hughes, et al., 1991). Increases are seen in respiratory rate, amplitude of reflexes, and the rate and force of the heart's contractions (systolic blood pressure). The

Caffeine Content		
SOURCE	SERVING	CAFFEINE(mg)
coffee (drip)	8 oz.	175–240
coffee (perked)	8 oz.	100–200
coffee (instant)	8 oz.	65–170
coffee (decaffeinated)	8 oz.	3–8
black tea (steeped 5 min.)	8 oz.	65–160
green tea (steeped 5 min.)	8 oz.	80
hot cocoa	8 oz.	3–16
cola beverages	12 oz.	45
"energy" beverages	8 oz.	80
milk chocolate	1 oz.	1–15
bittersweet chocolate	1 oz.	3–35
chocolate cake	1 slice	20–30
Anacin, Midol	2 tablets	64
Excedrin	2 tablets	130
NoDoz	2 tablets	200
Dexatrim	2 tablets	200

* Food & beverage contents approximate. Table 6.1

stimulating effects of caffeine can take up to 12 hours to wear off. Caffeine use contributes significantly to problems with sleep.

Caffeine causes a general *vasodilatation* (opening) of the systemic blood vessels, including the coronary arteries, resulting in an increase in blood flow to the heart. The duration of systemic vasodilatation is brief and is accompanied by a *vasoconstriction* (tightening) of the vessels in the brain (Hughes, et al., 1991). Central vasoconstriction is the mechanism by which caffeine provides relief from both hypertensive and migraine headaches. This is another reason why caffeine is often found in headache remedies.

Caffeine dependence

People who are caffeine-dependent have a strong association between caffeine consumption and feelings of well-being. Many people enjoy the increased speed of performance and feelings of efficiency and mental clarity caused by caffeine. Regular caffeine consumption causes both psychological dependence and physiological tolerance (Hughes, et al., 1991).

Caffeinism

This disorder is a chronic toxicity caused by very high levels of caffeine consumption. It is characterized by:

- disruption of sleep patterns
- nausea
- diarrhea
- headache
- trembling
- dry mouth
- rapid changes in mood
- depression
- stomach pain
- feelings of anxiety
- ringing in the ears
- irregular heartbeat
- palpitations

Caffeine withdrawal

The main symptom of caffeine withdrawal is headaches; if no caffeine is consumed these may continue for up to five days. The headaches often lead to use of analgesic preparations which may contain caffeine. This will cure the headache but lead to a continuance of caffeine dependence. Other symptoms of withdrawal are:

- apathy
- irritability
- restlessness
- decreased efficiency
- lethargy
- mild nausea
- nervousness
- difficulty concentrating

It is possible to reduce withdrawal symptoms by gradually decreasing the daily intake of caffeine by substituting decaffeinated coffee or tea and increasing the percentage of decaf each day.

Other Effects of Caffeine, Pros and Cons

Liver cancer

A study of more than 90,000 Japanese found that those who drank coffee every day, or nearly every day, had approximately half of the risk of contracting liver cancer than people who never drank coffee. The effect was seen in people who drank one to two cups of coffee per day and increased at three to four cups. This study was done at the National Cancer Center in Tokyo and was reported in the *Journal of the National Cancer Institute*. There was no association found between drinking green tea and liver cancer rates (Inoue, 2005)

Diabetes

One study that looked at the amount of coffee and tea consumed by 126,000 people over a 12-18 year period found that drinking more than four cups of caffeinated coffee per day reduced the risk of type 2 diabetes in men by about 50% and in women by about 30%. Drinking decaf resulted in a more modest effect, a 25% reduction in men and 15% in women. These data suggest that long-term coffee consumption is associated with a statistically significantly lower risk for type 2 diabetes (Salazar-Martinez, et al., 2004).

Heart disease and inflammatory disease

A fifteen year-long study was done with 27,312 women ages 55-69 who had not been diagnosed with heart disease, diabetes or cancer. Women who drank one to three cups of coffee daily were 24% less likely to die of heart disease compared with those who did not drink coffee. The coffee drinkers were also 28% less likely to die of other non-cancerous inflammatory diseases. Cancer deaths did not show any correlation with coffee consumption (Anderson, 2006).

Caffeine and cognitive decline

A study of cognitive decline looked at 4,179 women and 2,820 men (mean age 74), all of whom did not have dementia. After four years, the men had a normal age-related decline, but the women who drank at least three cups of coffee per day did not have a decline in verbal and visio-spatial memory. The overall risk of dementia was not related to the amount of caffeine consumed (Ritchie, et al., 2007).

Birth defects

Even though no significant correlation between birth defects and caffeine consumption has been demonstrated (Browne, 2006), it is important for women to know that caffeine crosses the placenta and gets into the bloodstream of a developing fetus. It also gets into the breast milk of nursing mothers. In both cases, the fetus or infant is ingesting a portion of the caffeine consumed by its mother.

Low birth weight infants

Maternal third-trimester serum paraxanthine concentration (which reflects caffeine consumption) was measured. Higher levels were associated with an increased risk of reduced fetal growth, particularly among women who smoked (Klebanoff et al., 2002).

Miscarriage

When pregnant women who did not consume caffeine were compared to pregnant women who did, the risk of miscarriage increased in direct proportion to the daily dose of caffeine consumed. In addition, the magnitude of the association appeared to be stronger among women without a history of miscarriage than among women with such a history (Weng, et al., 2008).

Bone loss

Daily consumption of more caffeine than the amount in about two to three servings of brewed coffee may accelerate bone loss from the spine and total body. This effect was seen only in women whose calcium intakes were below the recommended daily allowance (RDA) of 800 mg (Harris & Dawson-Hughes, 1994).

Fibrocystic breast disease

There seems to be a relationship between caffeine and *fibrocystic breast disease*. The specifics are not yet clearly understood (Hughes, et al., 1991). Decreasing caffeine consumption leads to a decrease in discomfort experienced by women with this disease. Although many studies have been done with large numbers of adults, and no correlation between caffeine consumption and breast cancer has been substantiated.

Effects of age and tobacco use on caffeine metabolism

A person's age will usually affect his or her physiological response to caffeine. Most people become more sensitive to caffeine's effects as they get older. It has also been observed that the amount of caffeine in the bloodstream increases when tobacco smoking is stopped. This increase in the blood level of caffeine can amplify the effects of nicotine withdrawal, such as irritability, nervousness, an inability to concentrate, and sleeplessness.

Anxiety

Studies show a positive correlation between caffeine use and anxiety disorders. People with anxiety disorders have an increased sensitivity to caffeine (Charney, et al., 1985). Symptoms of anxiety decrease with caffeine abstention, and for some people antianxiety medication is not necessary if caffeine use is discontinued (Bruce & Lader, 1989). The psychotherapist needs to assess caffeine intake in any patient who presents with symptoms of anxiety. In some individuals, reducing caffeine intake will eliminate the anxiety.

NICOTINE

The source of nicotine is the tobacco plant, *Nicotiana tabacum,* which is native to the western hemisphere. Tobacco was in use by indigenous peoples when the first explorers arrived from Europe, and its use quickly spread to the Old World (Borio, 2003). Today, nicotine is widely used in almost every country.

According to the Center for Disease Control and Prevention's 2004 report, about 23% of American adults (about 50 million people) use tobacco products. Although nicotine is extremely addictive and known to be harmful, its purchase and use by anyone over the age of 18 is legal. If one considers how difficult it is to stop using it, nicotine is even more addictive than opioids. Using nicotine, particularly through smoking, is much more harmful than using many other legal drugs in terms of the number of illnesses smoking causes, the costs of treating those illnesses, and the high fatality rates among habitual users.

Antismoking campaigns in the U.S. have lowered smoking rates, but there has been an increase in the percentage of people worldwide who smoke. It is estimated there are more than 440,000 smoking-related deaths every year in the U.S. alone (Longley, 2005). Although nicotine is the ingredient that causes physical dependency, it is the "tars" (the resinous, partially-combusted particulate matter produced by the burning of tobacco) that contain most carcinogens.

Nicotine and mood

Nicotine consumption causes the release of norepinephrine, dopamine, and serotonin in the CNS. This leads to feelings of both stimulation and decreased reactivity. Research indicates that part of the calming effect smokers experience is due to the decrease in the unpleasant withdrawal symptoms habitual users experience as nicotine levels in the blood drop. When nonsmokers or former smokers are compared to current smokers, indications are that nicotine is not calming but is actually a stimulant (Parrott, 1999).

It is now thought that nicotine withdrawal itself does not increase baseline anxiety. Rather, it is the response to stressors during withdrawal that is heightened (Jonkman, et al., 2008). This research supports the belief that relapse of smoking behaviors will be greater in people who are subjected to greater external stress. It follows that calming activities like meditation and yoga may support abstinence from nicotine.

Nicotine addiction and major mental illnesses

The release of DA is probably what leads to the reinforcing experience of pleasure associated with tobacco use (this release of DA is similar to that observed with other addictive drugs). Nicotine has a half-life of 30 minutes, which leads to an urge to consume more nicotine every half hour. Two cigarettes an hour (or the equivalent form of other tobacco products) will maintain a constant level of nicotine in the blood.

For reasons that are not yet clear, about 10% of smokers do not become addicted. They are able to keep consumption of cigarettes to approximately five per day, as opposed to the one or two packs a day consumed by the addict (Breslau, et al., 1991).

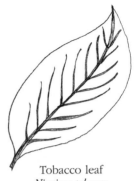

Tobacco leaf
Nicotiana tabacum

Recent research on cocaine may help to explain why some people become addicted to nicotine while others do not (Lohoff, et al., 2008). Genetic differences have been found between people who become dependent upon cocaine and those who remain casual users. Results suggest that variation in an enzyme, catechol-O-methyl transferase (COMT), which breaks down NE, 5-HT and DA, is related to the risk of dependency (Lohoff, et al., 2008). Similarly, genetic differences may explain why some people become dependant on nicotine.

People addicted to nicotine have higher rates of major depression and anxiety disorders than those who smoke but are not addicted (Walton, et al., 2001). One study found that 90% of people who attempt suicide are smokers (Leistikow, et al., 1996). More research is needed to analyze the factors responsible for these findings.

It is estimated that about 70% of people with schizophrenia smoke, a much higher percentage than in the general population. There is evidence that cigarette smoking ameliorates the unpleasant symptoms caused by schizophrenia and by antipsychotic medication. The harm-reduction approach combined with the nicotine patch or nicotine gum, is the recommended treatment for decreasing smoking in this population (McChargue, et al., 2003).

Smoking associated with cognitive decline

Using the Mini-Mental Status Exam, researchers examined changes in cognition over 2 1/2 years in 9,209 people over age 65 who did not have dementia. They found that a higher pack-per-year smoking exposure was associated with a greater decline in cognition (Ott, et al., 2004).

Tars & other compounds found in tobacco products

Some known carcinogens found in tobacco tars include:

- benzopyrenes
- aromatic amines
- pyrenes
- chrysenes
- nitrosamines

There are many other substances known to be harmful to humans that are frequently present in tobacco products, including:

- cresols
- phenols
- metallic ions
- radioactive compounds
- carboxylic acids
- various additives and flavoring agents
- agricultural compounds (e.g., pesticides)

If manufacturers removed these toxic agents from their products the harmful effects of tobacco use would be greatly reduced.

Nicotine withdrawal

Physiological symptoms of withdrawal occur when someone who is addicted to nicotine stops consuming it. This withdrawal syndrome is commonly called a "nicotine fit." Symptoms of withdrawal are:

- anxiety
- restlessness
- feelings of uneasiness
- headache
- nervousness
- digestive disturbances
- impairment of psychomotor performance
- impairment of concentration and judgement

When the body is under stress, nicotine is depleted faster than usual, causing the addict to increase consumption in order to maintain the usual blood-level of nicotine and prevent withdrawal symptoms.

TREATMENTS FOR NICOTINE WITHDRAWAL

Patches, gums, lozenges & inhalers for nicotine withdrawal

The nicotine patch, nicotine gum, nicotine lozenges, or a nicotine inhaler are all useful for helping people to decrease and quit tobacco use. Simply trying to "cut down" on smoking continues to expose the individual to the health risks and reinforcing behaviors inherent in tobacco use. These products all contain nicotine and are addictive but decrease the major health risks caused by inhaling smoke and permit tapered nicotine withdrawal. They also help to break behavioral patterns associated with tobacco use.

Bupropion & naltrexone for nicotine withdrawal

The FDA's Drug Abuse Advisory Council found that the antidepressant bupropion/Wellbutrin/Zyban is safe and effective as an aid in smoking cessation (Jorenby, et al., 1999). Another drug, naltrexone/Revia (developed for use during opioid withdrawal), has been found to decrease the craving for nicotine (Ahmadi, et al., 2003). Both of these drugs are useful as supportive measures in addition to psychotherapy, especially in the early stages of abstinence.

Varenicline tartrate

Varenicline/Chantix was approved by the FDA as an aid to smoking cessation treatment in May 2006. It is believed to work by blocking the stimulating and dopamine-releasing effects that occur when nicotine is consumed (Naiura, et al., 2006).

Black box warning

In 2008, the FDA announced that the connection between Chantix and serious psychiatric problems was increasingly likely. In 2009, the agency required that Chantix and another smoking-cessation drug, Zyban, carry the FDA's strongest safety warning regarding possible side effects (including depression and suicidal thoughts).

Clonidine for nicotine withdrawal

Another drug that may be helpful during nicotine withdrawal is clonidine/Catapres. Clonidine is an antihypertensive drug that has shown evidence of decreasing cravings during nicotine withdrawal (Ahmadi, et al., 2003; Gourlay, et al., 1994). Clonidine is not FDA-approved as a treatment for nicotine withdrawal.

Nicotine vaccine

The effect of immunization against nicotine was studied in anesthetized rats (Hieda, et al., 1999). Results found nicotine-specific antibodies and a reduction of the nicotine in the brain. These data suggested that the use of immunization of humans to modify the effects of nicotine may be possible.

Nic Vax (a nicotine vaccine) is now in Phase III human trials, and so far it seems to be both safe and effective, although the response rates seen are not better than those achieved by other available methods. This research suggests that the vaccine may be more useful for preventing relapse rather than for smoking cessation (Hatsukami, et al., 2005).

Effect of caffeine during nicotine withdrawal

Caffeine is metabolized more quickly by smokers than by nonsmokers. If someone stops using nicotine, and the amount of caffeine consumed remains constant, the level of caffeine in the blood will double. This will cause an increase in nervousness that makes withdrawal from nicotine even more difficult. For this reason, it is recommended that caffeine consumption be decreased or eliminated during withdrawal from nicotine (Bruce & Lader, 1989).

Attention Deficit Hyperactivity Disorder (ADHD)

Using the *DSM* definition, the prevalence of attention deficit hyperactivity disorder (ADHD) in the U.S. is between 8% and 16%. Boys are four times more likely to be given this diagnosis than are girls (Wender, 2002). Although there is much overlap between the symptoms of ADHD and childhood bipolar disorder, one difference is that children with ADHD still have a normal need for sleep, whereas children with bipolar disorder will not require normal amounts of sleep (John Preston, MD, personal communication, 8/26/06).

Genetic findings

There is strong evidence for a genetic component in ADHD. Twin studies show a 65-95% concordance rate. This is comparable to rates in schizophrenia and bipolar disorder (Brown, 2003).

Anatomical differences in brain scans of children with ADHD

Anatomical differences have been found in scans of areas of the brain which control communication in children diagnosed with ADHD. They found that these differences diminished in children who had been medicated with stimulant drugs for an average of 2 1/2 years (Ashtari & Kumra, 2004).

TREATMENTS FOR ADHD

Amphetamines & methylphenidate

Methylphenidate was synthesized in the 1940s and marketed under the brand name Ritalin in the 1960s (History of methylphenidate, 2003). In the U.S. alone, about 11 million prescriptions are written every year for methylphenidate (now including Concerta and Focalin) and another six million are written for various amphetamine compounds such as Adderall (DEA Congressional Testimony, 2000). These drugs are useful in decreasing hyperactive behavior in both children and adults. The mechanism for the paradoxical response in these populations (i.e., why taking a stimulant results in calming) is not yet fully understood (Gainetdinov, et al., 1999).

When taking methylphenidate, children who were previously unable to concentrate and had difficulty learning were able to perform at their age-appropriate level. Tolerance and dependence do not develop in children who are taking these medications. A slowing of growth has been observed when children take methylphenidate for long periods. This may be due to the appetite-suppressing side effect. To remedy this, children are given "drug vacations" from their medication on weekends and/or over the summer when they are not in school. This break usually allows children time to catch up on their growth if it had slowed due to the medication.

Methylphenidate and amphetamine can be drugs of abuse. They can be snorted or dissolved and then injected for a rapid effect (drug "rush"). When used in this manner, they have effects like cocaine, but milder. A tolerance will develop if they are used frequently in this way, and withdrawal symptoms will occur if one stops taking the drug (Chiang & Goldfrank, 1990).

Lisdexamfetamine dimesylate

Because of problems of abuse, a new formulation called a "prodrug" has been developed for the treatment of ADHD. This prodrug, lisdexamfetamine dimesylate/Vyvanse, is converted to an active compound in the liver. Because it does not become active until it is metabolized, it is less likely to be abused.

Guanfacine

Guanfacine/Intuniv was approved by the FDA in September 2009 for the treatment of ADHD in children and adolescents ages six to 17. It is thought to work by engaging NE receptors in the prefrontal cortex to improve memory, attention regulation, impulse control, and to decrease susceptibility to distraction (Waknine, 2009).

Atomoxetine

The drug atomoxetine/Strattera is the only FDA-approved treatment for ADHD in adults as well as in children. This drug is not officially considered a stimulant because it is believed to work more on NE than DA. For this reason it is not a controlled substance, so more doctors are willing to prescribe it. A major advantage of this medication is that it only needs to be taken once in the morning and its effect lasts until evening without causing insomnia. A 13-item diary was developed by the manufacturer so that parents could assess efficacy of the drug on their children. The symptoms evaluated included:

- oppositionality
- hyperactivity/impulsivity
- inattentiveness/distractibility
- inability to concentrate on structured tasks

Children were rated during the early morning and in the evening. According to parent ratings, atomoxetine was found to be effective in alleviating these symptoms (Michaelson, et al., 2003).

There are indications that reducing the dose of atomoxetine may be necessary for patients with impaired liver functions (Chalon, 2003). The FDA now requires a "black box" warning for this drug. The warning states that atomoxetine may increase the incidence of suicidal thinking in children and adolescents.

Cardiac risks with stimulants

In 2008, the American Heart Association issued guidelines recommending an electrocardiogram (ECG) as part of the medical workup for children and adolescents before starting them on ADHD medication. The American Academy of Pediatrics responded that there was no evidence that doing this would balance issues of risk, benefit, and cost-effectiveness in identifying risk factors for sudden death in children being treated with stimulants; therefore, an ECG was not warranted. The consensus reached was to call for "careful assessment" for heart conditions in children being considered for ADHD medication. This would include a physical examination and an in-depth family history to assess for risk factors and cardiac problems. The child's physician would then determine whether an ECG was appropriate. The risk of sudden cardiac death from these medications is about the same as the risk from participating in strenuous exercise (American Academy of Pediatrics, 2008).

Buspirone

Although developed as an antianxiety medication and not considered a stimulant, buspirone/Buspar has been found to be as effective as methylphenidate/Ritalin in reducing symptoms of ADHD, with minimal adverse effects. Some children experienced dizziness during the first week on buspirone (Malhotra & Santosh, 1998).

Caffeine & ADHD

Caffeine has been shown to improve functioning and reduce levels of hyperactivity in children with ADHD. Although traditional treatments with methylphenidate and amphetamines outperform caffeine in improving functioning, caffeine outperforms the control

groups getting no treatment. Some improvements are:
- better relationships with parents and teachers
- reduced aggression   • improved executive functioning
- reduced hyperactivity   • reduced impulsiveness (Chalon, 2003)

This evidence indicates that caffeine is helpful for children with ADHD and may be valuable as an alternative to the more potent stimulants (O'Connor, 2001). Opinions differ on whether caffeine use in children is harmful. No long-term studies have been done to assess its effects on physical and psychological functioning in children. Most children respond to caffeine in the same way as adults. There is a stimulating effect, observed as nervousness, and when tested, response time is shortened (O'Connor, 2001).

Caffeine may be an option for parents who are opposed to the use of other stimulants. This may ease their fears of the adverse effects on their children from the long-term use of more powerful stimulants.

ADHD and substance abuse

Parents are frequently concerned that treating their children with stimulants will increase the risk of substance abuse in the future. Many studies have been done to investigate this issue. In a meta-analysis of results from six studies where subjects were followed from four years old to adolescence and then to young adulthood, it was found that the risk of substance abuse was about half for the youths who were treated with stimulants as compared to youths who were not medicated for their ADHD. The risk reduction was similar when both alcohol abuse and drug abuse were evaluated (Wagner, 2004).

Stimulants for Treatment of Depression

The amphetamines and methylphenidate may be appropriate for short-term use to treat depression, but due to fears of their addictive potential, they are not frequently prescribed (Wagner, et al., 1997). Even the caffeine in coffee and tea will usually improve mood.

Stimulants can be useful for treating depression when apathy and lack of motivation are present. These drugs can help to get someone launched on a regime of exercise and constructive activities that may help to maintain an elevated mood. Their virtue is that as stimulants they act immediately, whereas most antidepressants take several weeks to reach their maximal effect. Immediacy can be critical if a patient is suicidal. It is this immediacy of response which also makes stimulants potential drugs of abuse. People who have no history of addiction usually do not become addicted when taking these drugs for therapeutic purposes (Satel & Nelson, 1989).

Direct Relevance to Psychotherapy

It is very important to be aware that a paranoid psychosis may result from long-term use of stimulant drugs (particularly with amphetamines or cocaine). This drug-related condition may be clinically indistinguishable from the paranoid psychosis seen with schizophrenia or during a manic episode. The symptoms may include: hostility, paranoia, delusions, aggressiveness, disorganized thought patterns, and hallucinations (usually auditory). These psychotic symptoms occur most often when there is a sudden increase in dosage, or in chronic users of amphetamines who are taking more than 100 mg/day.

The treatment of choice for this drug-induced psychosis is to stop using the stimulant and begin a course of antipsychotic medication. Recovery from a drug-induced psychosis is not always immediate; it may take days or weeks to clear. In some cases, the psychosis may last for years and require continuing the antipsychotic medication. Autopsy results show that heavy amphetamine use can cause permanent brain damage (Eisch, et al., 1998).

Each therapist's own history and personal experiences with smoking and other forms of tobacco use, and the diseases they cause, will strongly influence his or her feelings about tobacco and its associated ills. There is no denying that tobacco use is a health hazard. Consumption of nicotine, like any other addictive drug or unhealthy habit, deserves exploration in therapy. For clients who want to stop, cognitive and behavioral interventions have proven to be most effective for changing habits. The psychotherapist can discuss with the client whether, in addition to psychotherapy, a nicotine substitute or a medication like bupropion or naltrexone might be beneficial. If medication is desired, an evaluation and prescription by a physician is necessary. Studies demonstrate that using a nicotine patch, in conjunction with bupropion, while continuing in therapy, leads to significantly higher long-term rates of smoking cessation than the use of any of these without psychotherapy (Jorenby, et al., 1999).

References for Chapter 6

Ahmadi J., Ashkani H., Ahmadi M. & Ahmadi N. (2003). Twenty-four week maintenance treatment of cigarette smoking with nicotine gum, clonidine and naltrexone. *J. Subst. Abuse Treat.* 24(3), –255.

Anderson, L. (2006). Heart disease, inflammatory disease and coffee consumption in post menopausal women. *Am. J. Clin. Nutrition,* 83, 1039-1046.

Ashtari, M. & Kumra, S. (2004). Annual Meeting of the Radiological Society of North America. November 28-December 3, 2004, Chicago, IL.

Borio, G. (2003). The History of Tobacco: Part 1. Retrieved December 7, 2003 from http://www.historian.org/bysubject/tobacco1.htm

Breslau, N., Kilbey, M. & Andreski, P. (1991). Nicotine dependence, major depression and anxiety in young adults. *Arch. Gen. Psychiatry,* 48, 1069–1074.

Brodie, J., Figueroa, E., Laska, E. & Dewey, S. (2005). Safety and efficacy of gamma-vinyl GABA (GVG) for the treatment of methamphetamine and/or cocaine dependence. *Synapse,* 50, 261-65.

Brown, K. (2003). New attention to ADHD genes. *Science,* 301, 160-61.

Browne, M. (2006). Maternal exposure to caffeine and risk of congenital anomalies: A systematic review. *Epidemiology,* 17(3), 324-31.

Bruce, M. & Lader, M. (1989). Caffeine abstention in the management of anxiety disorders. *Psychological Medicine,* 19, 221–214.

Carpenter, S. (2001). Mixing medication and psychosocial therapy for alcoholism. *Monitor on Psychology,* June, 36–37.

Chalon, S. (2003). Hepatic impairment with atomoxetine. *Clin. Pharmacol. Ther.,* 73, 178–191.

Charney, G., Henninger, G. & Jatlow, P. (1985). Increased anxiogenic effects of caffeine in panic disorders. *Archives of General Psychiatry,* 42, 233–243.

Chiang, W. & Goldfrank, L. (1990). Substance withdrawal. *Emergency Medicine Clinics of North America,* Aug., 8(3), 613–614.

The coffee plant: Tree to cup/Harvesting. Retrieved December 7, 2003 from http://www.realcoffee.co.uk/Article.asp?Cat=TreeToCup&Page=1

Dackis, C., Kampman, K. & Lynch, K. (2005). A double-blind, placebo-controlled trial of modafinil for cocaine dependence. *Neuropsychopharm.,* 30, 205-11.

Dackis, C., Kampman, K., Pettinati, H. & O'brien, C. (2003). Effect of modafinil on cocaine abstinence and treatment retention in cocaine dependence: Preliminary results from open-label study. American Psychiatric Assn. 156th Annual Meeting. Abstract S&CR1-4. San Francisco, CA.

DEA Congressional Testimony, Caucus on International Narcotics Control, July 25, 2000, Fiano, R. A. U.S. Dept. of Justice, Drug Enforcement Administration.

Eisch, A., Schmued, L. & Marshall, J. (1998). Characterizing cortical neuron injury with fluro-jade labeling after a neurotoxic regimen of methamphetamine. *Synapse,* 3, 329.

Elkashef, A., Rawson, R., Anderson, A., Li, S., Holmes, T., Smith, E., Chiang, N., Kahn, R., Vocci, F., Ling, W., Pearce, VJ., McCann, M., Campbell, J., Gorodetzky, C., Haning, W., Carlton, B., Mawhinney, J. & Weis, D. (2008). Bupropion for the treatment of methamphetamine dependence. *Neuropsychopharm.,* 33(5), 1162-170.

Foxhall, K. (2001). Preventing Relapse. *Monitor on Psychology,* June 46–47.

Gainetdinov, R., Wetsel, W., Jones, S., Levin, E., Jaber, M. & Caron, M. (1999). Role of serotonin in the paradoxical calming effect of psychostimulants on hyperactivity. *Science,* 283(5400), 397–401.

Gerasimov, M., Schiffer, W., Brodie, J., Lennon, I., Taylor, S. & Dewey, S. (2000). Gamma-aminobutyric acid mimetic drugs differentially inhibit the dopaminergic response to cocaine. *Eur. J. Pharmacol.,* 395(2), 129–135.

Gibbs, J., Sombati, S., DeLorenzo, R. & Coulter, D. (2000). Cellular actions of topiramate: Blockade of kainate-evoked inward currents in cultured hippocampal neurons. *Epilepsia,* (Suppl. 1).

Golender, L., Bouquet. (2003). History of Tea: Botanics. Retrieved January 1, 2010 from http://www.gol27.com/HistoryTeaBotanics.html

Gourlay, S., Forbes, A., Marriner, T., Kutin, J. & McNeil, J. (1994). A placebo-controlled study of three clonidine doses for smoking cessation. *Clin. Pharma. and Therap.,* 55, 64–69.

Harris, S. & Dawson-Hughes, B. (1994). Caffeine and bone loss in healthy postmenopausal women. *American Journal of Clinical Nutrition,* 60, 573-578.

Hatsukami, D., Rennard, S., Jorenby, D. & Fiore, M. (2005). Safety and immunogenicity of a nicotine conjugate vaccine in current smokers. *Clin. Pharma. & Therap.,* 78, 456–467.

Hieda, Y., Keyler, D., Van DeVoort, J., Niedbala, R., Raphael, D., Ross, C. & Pentel, P. (1999). Immunization of rats reduces nicotine distribution to brain. *Psychopharmacol.,* 143, (2), 150-57.

History of methylphenidate. Retrieved December 7, 2003 from http://www.repsych.ac.uk/traindev/epd/adhd/drug/mpd1.htm

Hughes, J., Higgins, S., Bickel, W., Hunt, W., Fenwick, J., Gulliver, S. & Mireault, G. (1991). Caffeine self-administration, withdrawal, and adverse effects among coffee drinkers. *Archives Gen. Psych.,* 48, 611–617.

Inoue, M. (2005). The Japanese study was funded by the Ministry of Health, Labor and Welfare of Japan. Retrieved January 1, 2010.

http://www.msnbc.msn.com/id/6975257/

Jonkman, S., Risbrough, V., Geyer, M. & Markou, A. (2008). Spontaneous nicotine withdrawal potentiates the effects of stress in rats. *Neuropsychopharm.*, 33, 2131-38.

Jorenby, G., Leischow, S., Nides, M., Rennard, S., Johnston, J., Hughes, A., Smith, S., Muramoto, M., Daughton, D., Doan, K., Fiore, M. & Baker, T. (1999). A control trial of sustained-release bupropion, a nicotine patch, or both for smoking cessation. *New England J. Med.*, 340, 685–691.

Kampman, K. (2005). New medications for the treatment of cocaine dependence. *Psychiatry MMC.*, 2(12), 44-48.

Klebanoff, M., Levine, R., Clemens, J. & Wilkins, D. (2002). Maternal serum caffeine metabolites and small-for-gestational age birth. *Am. J. Epidemiol.*, 155(1), 32-37.

Krol, C. (2003). The coca plant. Retrieved December 7, 2003 from http://www.siu.edu/~ebl/leaflets/coca2.htm

Kuzniecky, R., Hetherington, H. & Ho, S. (1998) Topiramate increases cerebral GABA in healthy humans. *Neurology*, 51, 627-29.

Leistikow, B., Martin, D., Jacobs, J. & Sherman, C. (1996). A meta-analysis of the prospective association between smoking and suicide. *J. Addictive Diseases*, 15, 141.

Lohoff, F., Weller, A., Bloch, P., Nall, A., Ferraro,T., Kampman, K., Pettinati, H., Horwith, G. & Pentel, P. (2008). Association between the catechol-O-methyltransferase Val158Met polymorphism and cocaine dependence. *Neuropsychopharm.*, 33(13),3078-84.

Longley, R. (2005). Smoking deaths cost U.S. $92 billion a year. Total costs, including health care, more than $167 billion yearly. Retrieved February 21, 2010 http://usgovinfo.about.com/od/medicalnews/a/smokingcosts.htm

Malhotra, S. & Santosh, P. (1998). An open clinical trial of buspirone in children with attention-deficit/hyperactivity disorder. *J. Am. Acad. Child Adolesc. Psychiatry*, 37, 364–371.

McChargue, D., Gulliver, S. & Hitsman, B. (2003). Applying a stepped-care reduction approach to smokers with schizophrenia. *Psychiatric Times*, Sept., 78.

McGiverny, W. & Crooks, G. (1984). The care of patients with severe chronic pain in terminal illness. *JAMA*, 251(9), 1182-188.

McGregor, C., White, J., Srisurapanont, M., Mitchell, A. & Wickes, W. (2005). Open-label pilot trials of mirtazapine and modafinil in in-patient methamphetamine withdrawal symptoms and sleep problems. *67th Annual Sci. Mtg. Coll. on Probs. of Drug Depend.*, Orlando, FL. June 18-23.

Methamphetamine information: History of methamphetamine. Retrieved December 7, 2003, from http://www.narconon.org/druginfo/methamphetamine_hist.html

Michaelson, D., Adler, L., Spencer, T., Reimherr, F., West, S., Allen, A., Wernicke, J., Dietrich, A. & Milton, D. (2003). Atomoxetine in adults with ADHD: Two randomized, placebo-controlled studies. *Biol. Psychiatry*, 53(2), 112–20.

Munro, C., McCaul, M., Wong, D., Oswald, L., Zhou, Y., Kuwabara, H., Choi, L.,

Brasic, J. & Wand, G. (2006). Sex differences in striatal dopamine release in healthy adults. *Biol. Psychiatry*, 15, 59(10), 966-74.

Naiura, R., Jones, C. & Kirkpatrick, P. (2006). Fresh from the pipeline: Varenicline. *Nature Reviews Drug Discovery*, 5, 537-538.

O'Connor, E. (2001). A slip into dangerous territory. *Monitor on Psychology*, June, 60-62.

Orson, F., Kinsey, B., Singh, R., Wu, Y., Gardner, T. & Kosten, T. (2008). Addiction Reviews, Substance abuse vaccines. *Annals of the New York Academy of Sciences*, 1141, 257-269.

Ott, A., Andersen, K., Dewey, M., Letenneur, L., Brayne, C., Copeland, J., Dartigues, J., Kragh–Sorensen, P, Lobo, A, Martinez–Lage, J., Stijnen, T., Hofman, A. & Launer, L. (2004). Effect of smoking on global cognitive function in non-demented elderly. *Neurology*, 62, 920-24.

Parrott, A. (1999). Does cigarette smoking cause stress? *Am. Psychologist*, 54(10), 817–820.

Peng, X-Q., Lia, X., Gilberta, J., Paka, A., Ashby, C., Jr., Brodiec, J., Deweyd, S., Gardnera, E. & Xia, Z-X. (2008). Gamma-vinyl GABA inhibits cocaine-triggered reinstatement of drug-seeking behavior in rats by a non-dopaminergic mechanism. *Drug and Alcohol Depen.*, 97(3), 216-25.

Petrakis, I., Carrol, K., Nich, C., Gordon, L., McCance-Katz, E., Frankforter, T. & Rounsaville, B. (2000). Disulfiram treatment for cocaine dependence in methadone-maintained opioid addicts. *Addiction*, 95(2), 219–228.

Petroff, O., Hyder, F., Mattson, R. & Rothman, D. (1999). Topiramate increases brain GABA, homocarnasine, and pyrrolidinone in patients with epilepsy. *Neurology*, 52, 473-78.

Raby, W. & Coomaraswamy, S. (2004). Gabapentin reduces cocaine use among addicts from a community clinic sample. *J. Clin. Psychiatry*, 65(1), 84–86.

Rawson, R. & Ling, W. (2007). Methamphetamine abuse: Consequences and treatment. *Psychiatric Times*, June, 25-27.

Ritchie, K., Carrière, I., de Mendona, A., Portet, F., Dartigues, J., Rouaud, O., Barberger-Gateau, P. & Ancelin, M. (2007). The neuroprotective effects of caffeine. A prospective population study (The Three City Study). *Neurol.*, 69, 536-45.

Salazar-Martinez, E., Willett, W., Ascherio, A., Manson, J., Leitzmann, M., Stampfer, M. & Hu, F. (2004). Coffee consumption and risk for Type 2 diabetes mellitus. *Annals of Internal Medicine*, 140,1-8.

Satel, S. & Nelson, J. (1989). No reports of addiction using stimulants under medical supervision. *J. Clin. Psychiatry*, 50(7), 241–249.

Stahl, S. (1999). Awakening to the psychopharmacology of sleep and arousal: Novel neurotransmitters and wake-promoting drugs. *J. Clin. Psychiatry*, 63(4), 339–402.

Sussman, E. (1997). Cocaine vaccine is almost ready for the market. *Psychopharmacol. Update*, 8(2), 1, 7.

Thompson, P., Hayashi,K., Simon, S., Geaga, J., Hong, M., Sui, Y., Lee, J., Toga, A., Ling, W. & London, E. (2004). Structural abnormalities in the brains of human subjects who use methamphetamine. *J. Neuroscience*, 24, 6028-36.

Wagner, J., Rabkin, J. & Rabkin, R. (1997). Dextroamphetamine as a treatment for depression and low energy in AIDS patients: A pilot study. *Psychosomatic Research,* April, 42(4), 407–411.

Wagner, K. (2004). Childhood ADHD and adolescent substance use. *Psychiatric Times.* April, 2004, 92.

Waknine, Y. (2009). Once-daily guanfacine approved to treat ADHD. *Medscape, Medical News.* Retrieved January 3, 2010 http://www.medscape.com/viewarticle/708380.

Walton, R., Johnstone, E. & Munafo, M. (2001). Genetic clues to the molecular basis of tobacco addiction and progress towards personalized therapy. *Trends Mol. Med.,* 7(2), 70–76.

Wender, E. (2002). Attention-deficit/hyperactivity disorder: Is it common? Is it overtreated? *Arch. Pediatr. Adolesc. Med.,* 156, 209–210.

Weng, X., Odouli, R. & Li, D. (2008). Maternal caffeine consumption during pregnancy and the risk of miscarriage: a prospective cohort study. *Am. J. Ob. & Gyn.,* 198(3), 279e1–279e8.

Chapter 7

Treatment of Psychotic Disorders

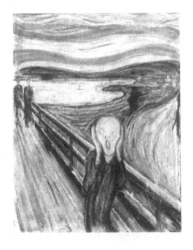

Since the 1940s, many drugs and other procedures, including insulin shock and ECT, have been effectively used to treat psychosis. Psychosis can be broadly defined as the loss of contact with reality (the presence of hallucinations and delusions). Although individual patients may respond to one drug better than another, to date it has not been demonstrated that any one drug is more effective overall than any other. One patient may respond well to a particular antipsychotic medication, but not to another, while a second patient, with a similar history and symptoms, may respond very differently. The drug clozapine deserves some further explanation with regard to effectiveness (see p. 133). There is currently no reliable method for predicting how any individual will react to any particular antipsychotic drug. Genetic analysis may change this in the future.

Psychoactive drugs are often selected based largely on their side-effect profile. For example, different antipsychotic drugs cause different levels of sedation, or cause differing amounts of weight gain, important factors in determining which to use. The psychiatrist, aware of these variables, evaluates which drug has the best chance of working and will have the fewest, and least dangerous, adverse effects for each individual patient.

Schizophrenia

About 1% of the population suffers from schizophrenia (Gottesman,

2001). There is strong evidence that this disease has a genetic component. Children of one schizophrenic parent have a 13% chance of becoming schizophrenic whether or not the child has been raised with the schizophrenic parent. There is a 48% concordance rate in monozygotic (identical) twins and a 13% rate in dizygotic (fraternal) twins. These statistics suggest the influence of both genetic and environmental factors in the occurrence of schizophrenia (Gottesman, 2001).

Positive & negative symptoms of schizophrenia

The symptoms of schizophrenia are characterized as either positive or negative. These terms do not indicate whether a symptom is "good" or "bad." Positive symptoms refer to things like hallucinations, hearing voices, and delusions that are present only in the patient's mind, whereas negative symptoms refer to the absence of some quality (e.g., turning inward, anhedonia, apathy, social withdrawal). New antipsychotic drugs are constantly being developed in the hopes that they will have fewer adverse effects and increased efficacy, in particular with regard to negative symptoms.

Antipsychotic Medications

Drugs used to treat psychotic symptoms have been called by many different names: major tranquilizers, phenothiazine tranquilizers, neuroleptics, and antipsychotic medications. To avoid confusion, the term "antipsychotic" will be used in this book to refer to all the drugs in this class. They will be categorized as: first generation antipsychotics (FGAs); second generation antipsychotics (SGAs); and one drug aripiprazole/Abilify, called a dopamine system stabilizer (DSS).

As the term antipsychotic indicates, this class of drugs is used for the treatment of psychoses. There are many disorders (e.g., bipolar mania, depression) and drug states (e.g., amphetamine and cocaine use, LSD) that may have psychotic symptoms. The medications in this chapter are used to treat psychotic symptoms regardless of the underlying cause.

When prescribed to treat a psychotic episode that is part of a depression or a bipolar disorder, these medications are usually taken on a short-term basis (four to five months). For a drug-induced psychosis (e.g., LSD or amphetamine) they may only be necessary for a few days, whereas with a diagnosis of schizophrenia they are generally taken over much longer periods, often for years.

Time-course for antipsychotic medications

When antipsychotic medication is started, there may be a period (sometimes as long as 12 weeks) of gradual improvement in psychotic symptoms (Wyatt, 1991). During this time, psychotherapy can consist of dealing with the practicalities of life and nurturing the development of a therapeutic alliance. A client who has psychotic symptoms often needs assistance and support getting along in the world on a day-to-day basis, this may include dealing with problems at work or school, learning to deal with family, and learning social skills. The therapist can help the client learn how to make simple decisions such as what type of milk to buy, as well as how to master complex tasks, like applying for a job, ways to become more self-sufficient and how to develop a healthy life style in general.

Optimal treatment for a client on medication requires a collaborative relationship between psychotherapist and psychiatrist. The psychotherapist sees the patient frequently, and may be the first to notice a disturbing adverse effect of a medication. If this occurs, a consultation with the psychiatrist is necessary to discuss the symptoms observed. The psychiatrist will then be the one to evaluate whether or not a serious condition is developing. Ongoing monitoring by the psychotherapist is important since some serious adverse effects (such as *tardive dyskinesia* or *neuroleptic malignant syndrome,* both discussed in this chapter) can emerge even after the patient has been on medication for a long period of time, sometimes years (Wyatt, 1991).

Effects of Antipsychotic Medications

There is evidence that psychotic symptoms are primarily caused by a disturbance in the DA system in the CNS. Put very simply, it is believed that, in schizophrenia, some parts of the brain have too little DA activity and other parts have too much. Antipsychotic medications attempt to correct these imbalances (Singh, et al., 1996).

The first effect seen when these drugs are started is sedation; the patient becomes calmer in several hours. This sedation is particularly valuable for treating manic patients, or for those who have violent, self-destructive, or suicidal ideation. Patients usually develop a tolerance to this effect in about two weeks. After several weeks, if the medication is working, patients report that their delusions, disordered thinking, and hallucinations either have disappeared, decreased, or that they are no longer as bothered by them.

Many patients with schizophrenia who are having a first psychotic episode and are put on medication will have a full remission of the hallucinations or delusions. If they stay on medication, the possibility of a relapse is greatly reduced but not eliminated (Wyatt, 1991). The relapse rate for patients maintained on antipsychotic medication is 15% to 30% in the first year, whereas patients who do not stay on medication have a relapse rate of 50% to 70%. Unfortunately, more than one-third of patients discontinue their medication due to adverse side effects, finances, or simply forgetting to refill the prescription. When medication is discontinued, at least 40% of patients have a relapse within six months (Wyatt, 1991).

No tolerance develops to the antipsychotic effect of these drugs and they do not cause euphoria, so there is no potential for abuse or addiction. There is evidence to suggest that repeated or prolonged psychotic episodes will gradually make the schizophrenic disorder worse. Patients may become discouraged and more socially isolated, and recovery often takes longer and becomes more difficult (Wyatt, 1991).

Studies show that psychotherapy without medication is no better than placebo for treating an acute psychosis. In other words, psychotherapy has no effect on the acute psychotic state. For long-term treatment, therapy and medication are better than medication alone. With schizophrenic patients, therapy helps most with improvement of social skills and social adjustment (Beers, et al., 2006).

First Generation Antipsychotics (FGAs)

This group, also called "typical" or "classical" antipsychotic drugs, has many specific adverse effects. Some of these occur less frequently with second generation antipsychotic (SGA) medications (see p. 133).

EXTRAPYRAMIDAL SYNDROME (EPS)

The most frequently seen adverse effects with FGAs are various movement disorders collectively called extrapyramidal syndrome (EPS). It is believed that EPS occurs when 78% or more of the DA receptors in the CNS are occupied with an antipsychotic medication (Beers, et al., 2006). Onset of EPS is clearly a dose-related effect and occurs in at least 10% of all patients on FGAs. Some EPS symptoms, particularly the presence of a tremor, resemble Parkinson's disease. Symptoms of EPS can last for several months. In contrast, these symptoms occur less frequently with the SGAs, and occur very infrequently with clozapine (Beers, et al., 2006).

Treatment of EPS with anticholinergic drugs

There has always been a question as to whether it is better to prescribe anticholinergic drugs to prevent EPS at the start of FGA medication or to wait for EPS to occur and then start on an anticholinergic medication. Some patients become very frightened and refuse to continue taking antipsychotic medication if EPS occurs. For this reason, many physicians will prescribe an anticholinergic medication, either trihexyphenidyl/Artane or benztropine/Cogentin, as a preventive measure before any symptoms of EPS appear. Others argue that because not all patients will get EPS, many do not need these extra medications since these drugs have their own adverse effects which must be weighed against their potential benefits (Beers, et al., 2006).

The anticholinergic drugs cause a decrease in the amount of ACh available to the neurons; this leads to decreased movement and a reversal of the EPS. These drugs also decrease anxiety and depression and may improve the negative symptoms of schizophrenia. Their adverse effects are:

- dry mouth
- nausea
- dizziness
- blurred near vision

The elderly, due to their already decreased levels of ACh (an effect of aging), may have more severe adverse effects, such as urinary retention and delirium (Beers, et al., 2006). It is now known that prolonged treatment with anticholinergic drugs to prevent EPS may increase the chance of developing TD.

Treatment of EPS with amantadine

Another drug sometimes used to treat EPS is the antiviral drug amantadine/Symmetrel, which increases DA activity. This will lead to a decrease in EPS. Adverse effects of amantadine include:

- dizziness
- insomnia
- seizures
- psychotic symptoms

TARDIVE DYSKINESIA (TD)

Tardive dyskinesia is a serious adverse effect caused by many FGAs. TD can appear at any time from three months to ten years after beginning medication. Frequently seen symptoms are:

- hand clenching
- finger movements such as choreiform (dance-like) movements
- oral and facial movements such as torticollis (tightening of neck and face muscles)

The rate of occurrence of TD in patients on FGA medications is 3% to 4% per year for the first five years. TD occurs most often in patients who have been maintained for many years on high doses of FGAs. As many as 50% of patients who were treated with these medications on a chronic basis (longer than five years) developed TD (Szymanski, et al., 1993). TD occurs with SGAs, but less frequently.

TD is reversible in more than 30% of patients who develop it if the antipsychotic medication is discontinued. For the rest, the TD does not remit even when medication is discontinued. TD does not respond to anticholinergic medication even though this is the usual treatment for movement disorders like EPS (Tamminga & Woerner, 2002).

Etiology of TD

The specific cause of TD is not fully understood. Many believe that TD is due to hypersensitivity and/or over-proliferation of dopamine receptors. Symptoms of TD can be temporarily diminished by increasing the dosage of antipsychotic medication, but over time this remedy will intensify symptoms. As scientific understanding of the complexity of the CNS and the various neurotransmitter and neuromodulator systems increases, so does the complexity of the various theories about the underlying mechanisms for tardive dyskinesia (Tamminga & Woerner, 2002).

Treatment of TD

Reserpine, lithium, vitamin B6, melatonin, ondansetron, or BzRAs sometimes are effective in alleviating TD (Sirota, et al., 2000). It is thought that Vitamin E may prove to be both prophylactic for TD and an effective treatment for TD (Zhang, et al., 2004). Reserpine depletes NE, DA, and 5-HT stores; when taken for two to four days it can relieve symptoms of TD, but may also cause a serious depression (Szymanski, et al., 1993). When TD occurs, most psychiatrists proceed by taking the patient off the causal antipsychotic medication and switching to clozapine or to one of the SGAs (if the patient is not already on one) since they cause a lower incidence of TD than the FGAs. It is thought that the newer drugs spend less time on the DA receptor, and for this reason they are less likely to cause movement disorders. As of this writing, there is no definitive, successful treatment for TD (Herzman, 2010).

Other adverse effects of antipsychotic medications

Frequently seen are:

- decreased appetite
- impotence in men
- infertility in women (decreased ovulation)
- decreased libido (decreased production of testosterone)
- decreased adaptability to external temperature changes

Antipsychotic drugs cause little or no respiratory depression. They do cause a decrease in seizure threshold, making the possibility of a seizure more likely. They can also cause:

- weight gain
- lactation (in men and women)
- impairment in liver function leading to jaundice
- formation of pigment deposits on the retina leading to impaired vision

NEUROLEPTIC MALIGNANT SYNDROME (NMS)

Neuroleptic malignant syndrome is a serious and sometimes fatal disorder caused by antipsychotic medications. The specific cause is thought to be the rapid blocking of a large number of DA r eceptors. Symptoms include:

- sweating
- altered mental state
- renal (kidney) failure
- high fever (up to 107°F)
- elevated white blood cell count
- increased pulse and respiration rate
- severe Parkinsonian muscle rigidity (can make walking or talking difficult or impossible)

NMS can occur when starting on a medication or when the patient has already been stabilized on it. It can appear in someone who in the past took antipsychotic medication without major problems, and then when restarted on the same drug, develops NMS. The syndrome develops quickly, over a period of 24 to 72 hours. NMS can persist from 10 to 14 days with shorter-acting preparations, or for as long as four weeks with the long-acting depot (see below) preparations.

Apomorphine, amantadine, bromocriptine, and L-dopa are sometimes helpful in alleviating NMS; this is probably due to their ability to cause an increase in dopamine activity in the CNS. ECT is also an effective treatment. The usual treatment regimen consists of discontinuing medication, hospitalization, and initiation of life-support measures (Strawn, et al, 2007). Estimates of the rate of occurrence of NMS range from 0.02% to 2.4% for all patients on antipsychotic medications. The fatality rate is high, approximately 10% (Ahuja & Cole, 2009).

Risk factors for NMS

Psychotherapists who are seeing patients who are taking antipsychotic medications need to know which patients are at the greatest risk of developing NMS. There are some clear indications as to who this will be. About 80% of affected patients are under age 40, and males are affected twice as often as females. There is also a direct correlation between the risk of getting NMS and a history of:

- psychomotor agitation
- higher doses of medication
- rapid increase in dose of medication
- high number of intramuscular medication injections (Viejo, et al., 2003)

Researchers have found that both the maximum amount of medication, and the total number of doses, were nine times greater in patients with NMS than in the control group (patients who did not get NMS). The mean number of intramuscular injections received was also nine times greater than that of the control group (Viejo, et al., 2003).

Intramuscular administration rapidly leads to very high levels of the antipsychotic drug in the blood-stream. This then leads to an abrupt blockade of DA activity in the CNS. This rapid blocking does not allow enough time for the body's compensatory mechanisms to maintain the homeostasis required for the life-support functions controlled by the CNS (Viejo, et al., 2003).

A common sequence of events for patients who develop NMS is this: A young male comes to an Emergency Room with symptoms of agitation and psychosis; he is given an injection of antipsychotic medication to rapidly calm him and to treat the psychotic symptoms. It is this rapid administration of a high dose of antipsychotic medication which seems to precipitate the NMS. If you are treating patients at a high risk for NMS, be sure they are informed of their risk. If any symptoms of NMS appear, the patient needs to be hospitalized and treated as soon as possible (Viejo, et al., 2003).

Depot preparations

In the 1960s some long-acting, injectable forms of antipsychotic medications called "depot" preparations were developed with the hope of improving patient compliance and thus reducing the rate of relapse and rehospitalization. In these long-acting preparations, the active drug is suspended in an inactive carrier and is administered via subcutaneous or intramuscular injection. The carrier causes the drug to be absorbed slowly; because of this the medication only needs to be administered every one or two weeks. The major problem with these preparations is that there is no way to quickly remove the drug from the body if adverse effects do occur. As a safeguard, patients are put on depot preparations only after a trial with a shorter-acting form of the same drug is seen to cause no adverse effects. There is no increased risk of NMS or TD with depot preparations as compared to oral forms of the same drug (Glazer & Kane, 1992).

With these preparations, the drug does not pass through the digestive tract to get into the bloodstream. Therefore, stable blood-levels are easier to maintain, the dose can be lower, and the side effects lessened compared to when the medication is taken orally. Many people dislike or are fearful of injections, so depot preparations are not widely used in the U.S. They are used primarily for patients who have compliance problems with oral medications or for people who don't like taking pills every day (Glazer & Kane, 1992).

Drug manufacturers are currently at work developing long-acting preparations of the SGAs. One such preparation is risperidone/Consta, designed to be injected and effective for two weeks; another is paliperidone/Invega, an oral extended-release form of risperidone.

Second Generation Antipsychotics (SGAs)

Manufacturers are continually developing new antipsychotic drugs with the hope of finding compounds that are effective in the treatment of the symptoms of schizophrenia but do not cause TD or other serious adverse effects. The newer drugs are called "second generation antipsychotics" (SGAs); this category includes the antipsychotics formerly called "atypical" or "novel." These agents act as antagonists at serotonin and other receptors, as well as at DA receptors. Current SGAs include: asenapine, clozapine, olanzapine, paliperidone, quetiapine, risperidone, and ziprasidone.

CLOZAPINE (THE ORIGINAL SGA)

Often considered in a class by itself, clozapine/Clozaril was the first of this group of drugs to be developed and was the model for those that followed. Introduced into clinical practice in Europe in 1975, it is used to treat psychoses, *Tourette's syndrome* (a disorder with symptoms of verbal and motor tics), and for the psychotic symptoms that are sometimes induced by the drug L-dopa (used to treat Parkinson's disease). Clozapine is unique in that it does not cause TD (Meltzer & Luchins, 1984), and for this reason it has been of great interest to researchers and drug companies, as well as to the patients who need to take antipsychotic medication and their families.

Adverse effects of clozapine

Clozapine produces minimal EPS and can even be used as a treatment for TD (Meltzer & Luchins, 1984). The reason it is not the first drug of choice for psychotic symptoms is that it can cause a serious, potentially life-threatening disorder called agranulocytosis (a blood disorder with a high fatality rate).

The incidence of agranulocytosis is approximately 1% to 2% for patients taking clozapine, a rate ten times higher than occurs with any other antipsychotic drug. The agranulocytosis can be reversed if clozapine treatment is stopped within two weeks of development of the disorder (Beers, et al., 2006). When on clozapine for the first six months, the patient's blood must be monitored on a weekly basis. If there are no signs of agranulocytosis, the frequency of the monitoring can be reduced to once every two weeks for the next six months, then to monthly for the rest of the time after that. The manufacturer will not supply clozapine if the monitoring is not done. Monitoring is required for as long as clozapine is taken.

Agranulocytosis seems to be an autoimmune response of the bone marrow to clozapine (Beers, et al., 2006). The peak for its occurrence is in the first four months of treatment, although cases have been reported throughout the first year. Because of the life-threatening nature of this adverse effect, clozapine is usually only given when patients have not responded to other antipsychotic medications. Thirty percent of patients who do not respond to other antipsychotic medications will respond to clozapine, although the first signs of improvement may not be seen for four to six months after the medication is started (Honigfeld, et al., 1984).

Other possible adverse effects of clozapine are:

- seizures
- sedation
- weight gain
- diabetes

- hypotension
- excessive salivation
- metabolic syndrome
- tachycardia (rapid heartbeat)

For some patients, clozapine causes a more noticeable improvement in social functioning than in psychotic symptoms (Meltzer, 1992). Improvement in social functioning is a rare and desirable outcome eagerly sought by manufacturers, doctors, and patients. Unfortunately, agranulocytosis can be life-threatening, and many patients refuse the required frequent blood draws. Some patients who have a very good response to clozapine will not tolerate the blood tests and therefore are not allowed to continue taking it.

Common Antipsychotic Medications

First Generation Antipsychotics (FGAs)

- chlorpromazine/Thorazine
- fluphenazine/Prolixin
- haloperidol/Haldol
- loxapine/Loxitane
- molindone/Moban
- perphenazine/Trilafon

Second Generation Antipsychotics (SGAs)

- amoxapine/Ascendin
- asenapine/Saphris
- clozapine/Clozaril
- olanzapine/Zyprexa
  Zydiss (soluble on tongue)
- paliperidone/Invega
- quetiapine/Seroquel
- risperidone/Risperdal/Consta
- ziprasidone/Geodon

Dopamine System Stabilizers (DSSs)

- aripiprazole/Abilify

Table 7.1

Other SGAs

Some newer antipsychotic medications have been developed with the hope of replicating clozapine's positive effects and elimination of its adverse effects. Among these are: asenapine/Saphris, olanzapine/Zyprexa, paliperidone/Invega, quetiapine/Seroquel, risperidone/Risperdal, and ziprasidone/Geodon. None of these is as effective as clozapine for people who have not responded to other antipsychotic drugs. They all cause a lower rate of EPS and TD than the FGAs, and they all claim to improve negative symptoms, but clozapine remains unique in its ability to prevent TD. Ziprasidone may cause some cognitive improvement when compared with other antipsychotic drugs (Harvey, et al., 2004). There is also evidence that olanzapine may be useful in the treatment of borderline personality disorder (Bogenschutz & Nurnberg, 2004).

Amoxapine as an atypical antipsychotic

Amoxapine/Asendin is an antidepressant medication that has effects similar to the antipsychotic drugs currently in use. Since it is already available as a generic drug it may be a viable low-cost alternative to the SGAs. Amoxapine has shown efficacy as an atypical antipsychotic in open trials. In a blind study comparing it to risperidone, amoxapine showed equivalent improvement in positive, negative, and depressive symptoms. Amoxapine was associated with fewer adverse effects than risperidone (Apiquian, et al., 2005).

Adverse effects of SGAs

There is strong evidence that taking most of the SGAs leads to impaired glucose metabolism which can cause weight gain, metabolic syndrome, and diabetes (Goldstein & Henderson, 2000). When on these medications patients need additional counseling about nutrition, exercise, hyperglycemia, and diabetes. The effect on glucose tolerance usually abates when the drug is stopped. Most of the SGAs cause significant weight gain. At the end of a five-year study of patients treated with clozapine, approximately 30% were diagnosed with type 2 diabetes. Diabetes was reported in 33% of patients taking olanzapine. Less change in weight has been attributed to ziprasidone. It is recommended that patients on SGAs be monitored for diabetes with a blood test every six months (Goldstein & Henderson, 2000; Newcomer, et al., 2002; Sernyak, et al., 2002).

Most of the SGAs have been reported to cause priapism (painful, prolonged erections). This can occur in men who are just starting on these medications and those who have been taking them a long time. The condition is a medical emergency as it can cause long-term serious consequences such as impotence, urinary retention, and gangrene. Most of the reported cases have been with patients taking risperidone, but the other antipsychotic medications, both FGAs and SGAs, and various other types of medications can also cause this disorder (Sood, et al., 2008).

Treatment of weight gain and metabolic syndrome

There is some evidence that nizatidine/Axid (used to treat ulcers) may decrease the amount of weight gained by patients taking olanzapine (an SGA) by 50%. There also has been some success using metformin (oral insulin used to treat type 2 diabetes) for weight loss with children who are taking SGAs (Cavazzoni, et al., 2003; Hinney et al., 2002; Morrison, et al., 2002).

Weight gain and clozapine

Clozapine is the antipsychotic drug that causes the greatest weight gain. Fluvoxamine/Luvox, if given with clozapine, attenuates weight gain. The fluvoxamine inhibits the metabolism of clozapine leading to higher blood levels at lower doses of clozapine. Patients receiving this combination had no significant change in body weight or body mass index (BMI) (Lu, et al., 2004).

Deaths with SGAs in elderly patients with behavioral disturbances

The FDA has determined that there is increased mortality in elderly patients with dementia who are treated with SGAs. A total of 5,106 patients were studied and an approximately 1.6-1.7 fold increase in mortality was found for patients who were taking SGAs as compared with placebo. Most of the deaths were due to heart-related events or pneumonia. There is now a black box warning on SGAs indicating this danger. The limited data available on FGAs (as to this adverse effect) suggests that they too may cause a similar increase in mortality (U.S. Food and Drug Administration Public Health Advisory, 2005).

Dopamine System Stabilizers (DSSs)

One of a newer group of antipsychotic drugs, dopamine-system-stabilizers (DSSs), is now on the market. The first (and so far only) drug in this group, aripiprazole/Abilify, is said to be useful for controlling both the positive and negative symptoms of schizophrenia. It seems to have fewer adverse effects than other antipsychotic medications. Most common adverse effects of aripiprazole are:

- nausea
- insomnia
- anxiety
- headache
- constipation

The manufacturer claims that its use will not lead to the weight gain and the development of diabetes seen with most SGAs.

Patients in a four-week trial who were given a combination of aripiprazole and olanzapine lost weight, had an improved lipid profile, and a decreased body mass index (Henderson, et al., 2009).

Selegiline augmentation for schizophrenia

Low doses of selegiline/Eldepryl (an MAOI) have been used to augment antipsychotic medications to treat the negative symptoms of schizophrenia. Patients who were taking antipsychotic medication for at least one year were given either selegiline or placebo in addition to their usual antipsychotic medications. There was significant improvement seen in the selegiline group and the drug appeared to be well tolerated by the subjects (Bodkin, et al., 2005).

Smoking and caffeine affect the metabolism of olanzapine and clozapine

Patients need to inform their psychiatrists if they change their intake of caffeine or nicotine. If taking olanzapine/Zyprexa or clozapine/Clozaril, their dose of medication may need to be adjusted (Pinninti, et al., 2005).

Sarcosine: an amino acid for schizophrenia

Taking sarcosine, a naturally occurring amino acid, can lead to improvement of symptoms of schizophrenia. Sarcosine is believed to work by blocking glycine reuptake; this leads to an activation of the NMDA receptor. Drugs that target this mechanism have been moderately successful in treating some symptoms of schizophrenia (Tsai, et al., 2004).

Dehydroepiandrosterone (DHEA) for the negative symptoms of schizophrenia

There has been little success to date using medications to treat the negative symptoms of schizophrenia such as anhedonia, flat affect, and social isolation. However, one study has shown that administering DHEA (see p. 203) to patients along with other antipsychotic medication led to a significant reduction in negative symptoms (Strous, 2003).

Nicotine analogs for cognitive deficits in schizophrenia

Some researchers theorize that the high rate of smoking in schizophrenic patients is a form of self-medication. This is the idea behind using nicotine analogs in treating patients with schizophrenia. The agonist drug, PHA-543.613, a nicotinic acetylcholine receptor (nAChR) agonist, shows promise as a treatment for impaired information-processing and cognitive deficits seen in schizophrenia, a problem that remains largely untreated (Smith, et al., 2006).

Estrogen therapy for schizophrenia

Australian researchers (Kulkarni et al., 2008) have found that adding transdermal estrogen (estradiol) for women on antipsychotic medications reduced their symptoms of schizophrenia to a significant degree. The study was 28 days long and used a control group of women who received antipsychotic medications alone. The researchers believe this is a promising new area to explore for future treatments of schizophrenia and other mental illnesses.

TMS for auditory hallucinations.

Patients who received 132 minutes of TMS (see Chapter 4) over nine days while taking antipsychotic medications showed a significant reduction in hallucinations compared to a control group. Half of these subjects had a return of their symptoms within 12 weeks, though some continued to have no hallucinations for up to one year. These researchers used MRI scans to determine which area of the brain is active when the patient is hallucinating, and then delivered stimulation to that area. This has helped 25% of patients whose hallucinations were not controlled by medications alone (Hoffman, et al., 2005)

An Alternative Treatment for Psychosis

Some valiant attempts have been made to treat psychotic patients in an environment where patients were not medicated and where there was round-the-clock care. One of these was Diabasis House, started in San Francisco in 1974 by John Perry. The design of the current U.S. health-care system does not support this type of intensive treatment, since a large number of people are needed to care for patients as they go through psychotic episodes (Cornwall, 2002). Because treatment settings like Diabasis House are very rare, therapists have few opportunities to explore the validity of these modes of treatment. For these reasons, use of antipsychotic medication is currently the primary method used to treat psychotic symptoms.

Direct Relevance to Psychotherapy

Most therapists agree it is difficult to do effective psychotherapy with a person who is delusional. It is important to first get the psychotic symptoms under control, usually with medication, and then proceed with psychotherapy to work on the negative symptoms (if present).

To understand how medications are most appropriately used in the treatment of schizophrenia, it is helpful to examine the symptoms in the categories of "positive" (more overt symptoms), and "negative" (less obvious, more asocial features). Negative symptoms usually increase over time, and positive symptoms usually decrease with or without treatment. Each person may experience different proportions of positive and negative symptoms throughout the course of the disease, and some individuals may experience more of one type of symptom than the other. Most antipsychotic medications treat the positive symptoms of schizophrenia, but do not have much, if any, influence on the negative symptoms. Psychotherapy can greatly impact negative symptoms, but usually does not have any impact on positive symptoms. Therefore, the combination of medication and psychotherapy is usually necessary to provide optimal treatment for patients with psychotic disorders, and for schizophrenia in particular.

References for Chapter 7

Ahuja, N. & Cole, A. (2009). Hyperthermia syndromes in psychiatry. *Adv. Psychiatr. Treat.,* 15, 181-191.

Apiquian, R., Fresan, A., Ulloa, R-E., de la Fuente-Sandova, C., Herrera-Estrella, M.,

Vazquez, A., Nicolini, H. & Kapur, S. (2005). Amoxapine as an atypical antipsychotic: A comparative study vs risperidone. *Neuropsychopharm.*, 30, 2236-244.

Beers, M., Porter, R. & Jones, T. (2006). *The Merck Manual of Diagnosis and Therapy, (18th ed.)*. Rahway, NJ: Merck, Sharp & Dohme Research Laboratories.

Bodkin, J., Siris, S., Bermanzohn, P., Hennen, J. & Cole, J. (2005). Double-blind, placebo-controlled, multicenter trial of selegiline augmentation of antipsychotic medication to treat negative symptoms in outpatients with schizophrenia. *Am. J. Psychiatry*, 162(2), 388-390.

Bogenschutz, M. & Nurnberg, G. (2004). Olanzapine vs. placebo in the treatment of borderline personality disorder. *J. Clin. Psychiatry*, 65(1), 104–109.

Cavazzoni, P., Tanaka, Y., Roychowdhury, S., Breier, A. & Allison, D. (2003). Nizatidine for prevention of weight gain with olanzapine: A double-blind placebo-controlled trial. *Eur. Neuropsychopharm.*, 13(2), 81–85.

Cornwall, M. (2002). Alternative treatment of psychosis: A qualitative study of Jungian medication-free treatment at Diabasis. Doctoral dissertation, CIIS, SF, CA.

Glazer, W. & Kane, J. (1992). Depot neuroleptic therapy: An underutilized treatment option. *J. Clin. Psychiatry*, 53, 426–433.

Goldstein, L. & Henderson, D. (2000). Atypical antipsychotic agents and diabetes mellitus. *Primary Psychiatry*, 7(5), 65–68.

Gottesman, I. (2001). Psychopathology through a life-span genetic perspective. *American Psychologist*, November, 867–878.

Harvey, P., Meltzer, H., Simpson, G., Potkin, S., Loebel, A., Siu, C. & Romano, S. (2004). Improvement in cognitive function following a switch to ziprasidone from conventional antipsychotics, olanzapine, or risperidone in outpatients with schizophrenia. *Schizophrenia Research*, 66(2–3), 101–113.

Henderson, D., Fan, X. & Copeland, P. (2009). Aripiprazole added to overweight and obese olanzapine treated schizophrenia patients. *J. Clin. Psychopharmacol.*, 29(4), 165-169.

Herzman, M. & Adler, L. (Eds.) (2010). *Clinical Trials in Psychopharmacology*, 2nd Edition. Oxford, England: Wiley Blackwell.

Hinney, A., Hoch, A., Geller, F., Schafer, H., Siegfried, W. & Goldschmidt, H. (2002). Ghrelin gene: Identification of missense variants and a frameshift mutation in extremely obese children and adolescents and healthy normal weight students. *J. Clin. Endricinol. Metab.*, 87, 2716.

Hoffman, R., Gueorguieva, R., Hawkins, K., Varanko, M., Boutros, N., Wu, Y., Carroll, K. & Krystal, J. (2005). Temporoparietal transcranial magnetic stimulation for auditory hallucinations: Safety, efficacy and moderators in a fifty patient sample. *Biol. Psychiatry*, 58(2), 97-104.

Honigfeld, G., Patin, J. & Singer, J. (1984). Clozapine: Antipsychotic activity in treatment-resistant schizophrenics. *Adv. Ther.*, 1(2), 77–79.

Kulkarni, J., de Castella, A., Fitzgerald, P., Gurvich, C., Bailey, M., Bartholomeusz, C. & Burger, H. (2008). Estrogen in severe mental illness: A potential new treatment approach. *Arch. Gen. Psychiatry*, 65(8), 955-960.

Lu, M., Lane, H., Lin, S., Chen, K. & Chang, W. (2004). Adjunctive fluvoxamine inhibits clozapine-related weight gain and metabolic disturbances. *J. Clin. Psychiatry*, 65, 766-771.

Meltzer, H. (1992). Dimensions of outcome with clozapine, *Brit. J. Psychiatry*, 160(Suppl. 17), 46–53.

Meltzer, H. & Luchins, D. (1984). Effect of clozapine in serve tardive dyskinesia: A case report. *J. Clin. Psychopharm.*, 4(5), 286–287.

Morrison, J., Cottingham, E. & Barton, B. (2002). Metformin for weight loss in pediatric patients taking psychotropic drugs. *Am. J. Psychiatry*, 159(4), 655-657.

Newcomer, J., Haupt, D. & Fucetola, R. (2002). Abnormalities in glucose regulation during antipsychotic treatment of schizophrenia. *Arch. Gen. Psychiatry*, 59, 337–345.

Pinninti, N., Mago, R. & de Leon, J. (2005). Coffee, cigarettes and meds: What are the metabolic effects? *Psychiatric Times*, May, 20-24.

Sernyak, M., Leslie, D., Alarcon, R., Losonczy, M. & Rosenheck, R. (2002). Association of diabetes mellitus with use of atypical neuroleptics in the treatment of schizophrenia. *Am. J. Psychiatry*, 159(4), 561–566.

Singh, A., Barlas, C., Singh, S., Franks, P. & Mishra, R. (1996). A neurochemical basis for the antipsychotic activity of loxapine: Interactions with dopamine D1, D2, D4 and serotonin 5-HT2 receptor subtypes. *J. Psychiatry Neurosci.*, 21(1), 29–35.

Sirota P., Mosheva, T., Shabtay, H., Giladi, N. & Korczyn, A. (2000). Use of the selective serotonin 3 receptor antagonist ondansetron in the treatment of neuroleptic-induced tardive dyskinesia. *Am. J. Psychiatry*, 157, 287–289.

Smith, R., Warner-Cohen, J., Matute, M., Butler, E., Kelly, E., Vaidhyanathaswamy, S. & Kahn, A. (2006). Effects of nicotine nasal spray on cognitive function in schizophrenia. *Neuropsychopharm.*, 31, 637-643.

Sood, S., James, W. & Bailon, M. (2008). Priapism associated with atypical antipsychotic medications: A review. *Int. Clin. Psychopharm.*, 23, 9-17.

Strous, R. (2003). DHEA augmentation for negative symptoms of schizophrenia, *Arch. Gen. Psychiatry*, 60, 133–141.

Strawn, J., Keck, P. & Caroff, S. (2007). Treatment in psychiatry: Neuroleptic malignant syndrome. *Am. J. Psychiatry* 164, 870-876.

Szymanski, S., Munne, R., Gordon, M. & Lieberman, J. (1993). A selective review of recent advances in the management of tardive dyskinesia. *Psych. Annals*, 23(4), 41–47.

Tamminga, C. & Woerner, M. (2002). Clinical course and cellular pathology of tardive dyskinesia. In: Davis, K., Charney,D., Coyle, J. & Nemeroff, C. (Eds.) *Neuropsychopharmacology: The Fifth Generation of Progress*. Philadelphia: Lippincott Williams & Wilkins. 1831–841.

Tsai, G., Lane, H., Yang, P., Chong, M. & Lange, N. (2004). Glycine transporter I inhibitor, N-methylglycine (sarcosine), added to antipsychotics for the treatment of schizophrenia. *Biol. Psychiatry*, 55(5), 452–456.

U.S. Food and Drug Administration Public Health Advisory. (2005). Deaths with SGAs in elderly patients with behavioral disturbances. RS-1659B.

Viejo, L., Morales, V., Punal, J. & Sancho, R. (2003). Risk factors in neuroleptic malignant syndrome. A case control study. *Acta. Psychiatr. Scand.*, 107, 45–49.

Wyatt, R. (1991). Neuroleptics and the natural course of schizophrenia. *Schizophrenia Bulletin*, 7(2), 325–351.

Zhang, X., Zhou, D., Cao, L., Xu, C., Chen, D. & Wu, G. (2004). The effect of vitamin E treatment on tardive dyskinesia and blood superoxide dismutase: A double-blind placebo controlled trial. *J. Clin. Psychopharmacol.*, 24(1), 83-86.

Chapter 8

Pain & Treatments of Pain

It is easier to find men who will volunteer to die than to find those who are willing to endure pain with patience.

Julius Caesar

Pain is one of the most common reasons people seek medical care, with headaches alone accounting for 45 million visits to the doctor in America each year (National Center for Health Statistics, 2007). One in every six Americans suffers from chronic pain. This number suggests that many people are taking over-the-counter or prescription pain medications. These medications often cause changes in consciousness, memory, and emotional state.

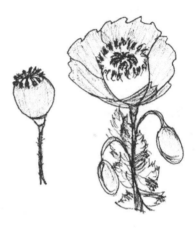

Opium poppy
Papaver somniferum

Certain types of pain can only be relieved by potent medications like morphine and other opioid-like compounds. Millions of people rely on these drugs in order to tolerate their pain and to have some semblance of a normal life. Pharmacologists have been trying for decades to develop a drug that alleviates deep pain but does not cause physical dependency. So far, they have not been successful.

SEROTONIN & THE PAIN RESPONSE

Serotonin (5-HT) is one of the many compounds that has a role in the pain response. When 5-HT is depleted, sensitivity to pain increases. The action of morphine on pain requires the presence of 5-HT. It has been shown that morphine's analgesic effect is blocked when serotonin is depleted (Ventafridda, et al., 1990).

Antidepressants, specifically duloxetine/Cymbalta and amitripty-line/Elavil, are helpful in alleviating certain types of pain, particularly migraine headaches, neurological pain, and the pain caused by fibromyalgia. This is probably due to their effect on serotonin levels. In the past, these types of pain could only be treated successfully with medications that could cause physical dependence.

The triptans, such as Imitrex and Treximet (a combination of sumatriptan and naproxen) are two medications used to treat migraine headaches. Both use the activation of the serotonin receptor as the mechanism for the pain relief.

Hierarchy of Treatment for Pain

There is a hierarchy in the treatment of pain based upon the side effects and addictive potential of the drugs used. Non-opioid drugs have what is called an "analgesic ceiling," the dose above which no further relief (analgesic effect) can be obtained. In general, opioids are used when pain cannot be adequately controlled using other treatments. For most opioids, there is no analgesic ceiling. The opioid dose can be increased until pain is relieved or until side effects become problematic. Because of variations in drug absorption, metabolism, tolerance and each individual's subjective experience of pain, there is no standard opioid dose (Ansari, 2000; Gatchel & Weisberg, 2000). Most doctors are reluctant to prescribe opioids due to their addictive potential and to their sedating and respiratory-depressant side effects (Joranson, et al., 1992).

Recent concerns about the adverse effects of NSAIDs, COX-2 inhibitors, and acetaminophen/Tylenol (specifically liver failure and an increased rate of cardiovascular problems for people who regularly drink alcohol), have caused physicians to reconsider using these medications as a first-line pain treatment (Griffin, 2005). Depending on an individual's risk factors, an opioid may be prescribed before a NSAID, COX-2 inhibitor, or acetaminophen. People with substance use

PAIN AND TREATMENTS OF PAIN | 145

disorders are at particularly high risk of experiencing these adverse effects. This presents a treatment dilemma since this is the population (those who regularly drink alcohol) which might have the most problems with opioids because of the potential for abuse.

ASPIRIN, NSAIDS, ACETAMINOPHEN, & COX-2 INHIBITORS

When someone is suffering from mild pain, the first drugs usually tried are aspirin and other over-the-counter preparations (e.g., Anacin, Excedrin, acetaminophen/Tylenol) or one of the nonsteroidal anti-inflammatory agents (NSAIDs) like ibuprofen/Motrin or naproxen/Aleve; these are most useful for treating pain resulting from inflammation. Adverse effects may include:

- increased clotting time
- gastric disturbances
- bleeding ulcers or severe irritation of the stomach

**Warning: These must be taken with food or a
full glass of water to avoid the stomach irritation.**

Because of their anticoagulant properties, NSAIDs should not be taken if there is heavy menstrual or other bleeding, or within three weeks of a surgical procedure. Acetaminophen is not an anti-inflammatory agent and it does not have anticoagulant properties. People frequently take it if they are allergic to aspirin or the NSAIDs. The cyclooxygenase-2 (COX-2) inhibitors such as celecoxib/Celebrex (available only by prescription) were developed to reduce the risk of stomach irritation caused by aspirin and the NSAIDs (Schlegel, 1987).

Corticosteroids

Corticosteroids (e.g., prednisone, cortisone) act as anti-inflammatory agents and are used when the non-steroidal anti-inflammatory drugs are not providing adequate relief. They are often administered by injection at the site of the pain for arthritic ailments such as back pain and bursitis. The most severe adverse effect of these drugs is that, if used frequently in this manner, they eventually can destroy bone (Leo, 2002). If taken systemically and long-term, they depress the immune system. Taken long-term, corticosteroids may cause specific psychological symptoms, usually manic episodes with psychotic features. Psychoactive medication may be required to treat these symptoms.

TRANSCUTANEOUS ELECTRICAL NERVE STIMULATION (TENS)

TENS is the administration of an electrical pulse directly at the site of the pain. The pulse is generated by a portable, battery-operated device, worn and controlled by the patient, who self-regulates the pulse as needed. TENS is often used for chronic pain (particularly back pain) when the pain is not very severe and the patient does not want to be constantly taking medication or have to deal with the adverse effects of drugs (Avellanosa & West, 1982). A semi-permanent, TENS-like device that is implanted into the spinal cord is now available.

ANTIDEPRESSANTS, ANTICONVULSANTS & OTHER DRUGS

Other medications are used alone or to augment the above treatments if they are inadequate. Many in the following list are discussed in detail elsewhere in this book.

- Anticonvulsant agents (e.g., topiramate) are useful for neuropathic pain and migraine prophylaxis.
- BzRAs (e.g., diazepam) are useful for muscle spasm relaxation and restless leg syndrome.
- Herbal agents (e.g., arnica, calendula) are useful for skin injuries and muscle pain.
- Lithium and topiramate are useful for cluster headaches.
- NMDA receptor blockers (e.g., ketamine, methadone) are useful for *post-herpetic neuralgia.*
- Stimulants are used to augment opioid narcotic agents.
- Topical agents (e.g., capsicum, lidocaine) are useful for arthritic pain.
- Triptans are useful for migraines (acute treatment).
- TCAs or SSRIs are useful for migraine headaches and fibromyalgia (prophylactic treatment).

OPIUM & OTHER NARCOTIC DRUGS

Opium is the finger of God. It smites, and it heals. It is the gift of heaven when it stills the agonies of death from cancer.

Harry Anslinger, Commissioner, Federal Bureau of Narcotics, 1930–1962

The class of drugs called opioids derives its name from the opium poppy, *Papaver somniferum*, which is native to the Middle East and has been known since ancient times for its strong narcotic effect. The poppy's seed capsule oozes a milky resin, which when collected and dried, becomes opium. Derivatives include morphine, heroin, and codeine. The opioids contain both natural and synthetic compounds that act on the body in similar ways. All of the opioids selectively bind to specific opioid receptors in the CNS, the GI tract, and the eye.

Opioid receptors in the CNS

Specific endogenous opioid receptors (different types with different behavioral effects) have been found in various parts of the brain. Opioids activate inhibitory pathways in the CNS. When these receptors are activated, either with an opioid or via TENS, the pain impulse is inhibited and analgesia results. Opioid receptors that appear to mediate deep pain have been identified; this pain is relieved by opioid narcotics but not by other types of pain medications.

Specific areas in the spinal cord are involved in the integration of incoming sensory information. If nerve cells in these areas are

---

Common Opioids

High Efficacy	Medium Efficacy	Low Efficacy
• diacetylmorphine/heroin	• buprenorphine/Subutex	• butorphanol/Stadol
• fentanyl/Sublimaze	• hydrocodone/Vicodin	• codeine
• hydromorphone/Dilaudid	• nalbuphine/Nubain	• pentazocine/Talwin
• meperidine/Demerol	• oxycodone/Percodan	• propoxyphene/Darvon
• methadone/Dolophine	• oxycodone HCl/OxyContin	
• morphine		
• oxymorphone HCl/Opana		

Table 8.1

inhibited, there is a decrease in painful stimuli transmitted from the spinal cord to the brain. Acupuncture may decrease pain through this mechanism (Avellanosa & West, 1982; Gol, 1967; Lazorthes et al., 1985; Mantyh, 2000).

The areas of the limbic system that are associated with emotional responses contain the greatest concentration of opioid receptors. The amygdala, an area of the brain that controls the anger response, is heavily innervated with opioid receptors. Since opioid systems are inhibitory, this inhibition could lead to a decrease in the pain of both physical and emotional stimuli (Gol, 1967).

Even though the treatment of severe or chronic pain presents many difficulties with regard to addiction and physical dependence, the opioids in their pure forms are very safe in terms of kidney, liver or stomach damage (Griffin, 2005). Opioids and other derivatives of opium are usually prescribed only when the milder forms of pain medications (see above) and TENS have not been adequate to control the pain. All currently-available opioid pain medications have many adverse effects, including:

- clouding of consciousness
- physical dependence • pupillary constriction
- constipation • loss of appetite • loss of sexual desire

Morphine

Morphine, the chief active ingredient of opium, has both sedative and analgesic properties. Its molecular structure resembles the endorphins (the main transmitter substances involved in the control of pain). Morphine enters the bloodstream in a water-soluble form and therefore cannot pass easily through the blood-brain barrier (see Appendix B). Due to its molecular structure, ten times more heroin than morphine is able to pass through the barrier and into the brain.

Tolerance, cross-tolerance, & overdose

Very large doses of any opioid will cause respiratory depression through inhibition of the respiratory center in the brain stem. Some tolerance to respiratory depression develops with opioids, unlike with barbiturates and alcohol, where little, if any, develops. Tolerance to the analgesic, euphoric, sedative, and emetic (induction of vomiting) effects of opioids develops over time. Very little tolerance develops to the antidiarrhea effect or the pupillary constriction. This is why the presence of "pin-point pupils" is diagnostic for opioid intoxication even in long-term users (Chiang & Goldfrank, 1990).

Cross-tolerance develops between different opioids, both natural and synthetic, even those that are chemically quite different. Cross-tolerance does not develop between opioids and barbiturates, alcohol, or sedative-hypnotic drugs. This lack of cross-tolerance is the main cause of many of the accidental deaths that result from combining these drugs. Combining sedatives or alcohol with an opioid can depress the respiratory centers to the point of causing coma and death.

All opioids are metabolized by the liver and excreted by the kidneys. Tolerance develops due to both an increase in synthesis of liver enzymes (see Appendix E) and to a decrease in sensitivity at the opioid receptors. A person suffering from liver or kidney disease has an impaired ability to metabolize opioids; this can lead to a drug accumulation that can reach toxic and overdose levels. Therefore, the risk of drug overdose is increased for anyone who has had hepatitis or any liver or kidney disease.

ADDICTION TO OPIOIDS

Most people become addicted to opioids due to a desire for euphoric feelings and/or a blunting of pain. Tolerance to the euphoric effect develops after only one week of daily use. When given morphine for medical purposes (usually every six hours for severe pain), patients develop some physical dependence after only two or three days. Addiction is rare after this brief treatment for severe pain, though when the drug is stopped mild withdrawal symptoms will be experienced. Most people (with no history of addiction) do not like the clouding of consciousness caused by narcotics and do not continue taking them once they can tolerate their pain using non-narcotic medications (Leo, 2002).

Physical dependence will always develop when opioids are taken for chronic and severe pain for long periods of time (weeks or months). In these situations, stopping the drug will be difficult and withdrawal symptoms will be more severe. Medical supervision or in-patient treatment for withdrawal can be helpful, but is not essential. Although the process of opioid withdrawal is extremely uncomfortable and unpleasant, it is not life-threatening (Chiang & Goldfrank, 1990).

Agonist & antagonist

An understanding of the terms "agonist" and "antagonist" is very important in comprehending how various drugs are used to treat opioid addiction, overdose, and withdrawal. (See Appendix D for a more detailed discussion of these terms.)

Treatment of opioid overdose

Opioid overdose is usually due to not knowing the exact dose of drug taken or one's level of tolerance. These circumstances are most apt to occur when drugs are obtained illegally. An overdose is usually treated in a hospital emergency room with the opioid antagonist naloxone/Narcan (see p. 151). Since naloxone is shorter-acting than most opioids, a patient who has overdosed needs to be hospitalized and observed for 24 to 48 hours so that the naloxone treatment can be repeated if necessary. If the patient is not monitored, the opioid antagonist may wear off before the opioid does, and respiratory depression may recur.

In conjunction with reversing the respiratory depression, opioid antagonists bring on symptoms of withdrawal. Severity of withdrawal symptoms is dependent upon many factors. Some of these are: the type of opiate used, the time since the last dose, the individual's degree of tolerance, and the individual's emotional reaction to the withdrawal symptoms (Chiang & Goldfrank, 1990).

Naloxone

Naloxone/Narcan is a pure narcotic antagonist; it has no opiate-like effects. It is used in emergency rooms in cases of overdose when rapid reversal of respiratory depression is necessary to save the person's life. Naloxone can be administered by intravenous injection, reaching the brain in about five minutes. It can also be administered by intramuscular or subcutaneous injection, which takes longer to take effect (Chiang & Goldfrank, 1990). It is not active if given orally.

Withdrawal symptoms will occur immediately if naloxone is injected into someone addicted to opiates.

Opioid-related deaths often involve use of multiple drugs, usually alcohol or a BzRA combined with the opioid. Taking an opioid with another drug that depresses respiration greatly increases the chance of death (Drake & Zador, 1996).

Treatment of addiction

There are many schools of thought on the best way to treat addiction. Some frequently-used therapies are:

- cognitive therapy
- behavior modification
- pharmacological interventions
- various combinations of all of these
- 12-step programs
- psychodynamic therapy

All of the methods listed above, alone or in combination, are successful for some people. It is important that the client be made aware of the various treatment options. Medications to ease the withdrawal symptoms can be helpful as adjuncts to psychotherapy. The therapist, client, and psychiatrist need to evaluate whether any of the drug therapies are desirable and appropriate. A few of the treatments for opioid addiction are discussed below.

OPIOID WITHDRAWAL & TREATMENTS

Withdrawal symptoms will begin 6 to 12 hours after the last dose (see Table 8.2, p. 153). They usually peak in 48 to 72 hours, then gradually lessen and disappear after 7 to 10 days. Withdrawal from opioids is not life-threatening, whereas withdrawal from barbiturates, the BzRAs, and alcohol can be (Chiang & Goldfrank, 1990). The protracted withdrawal period often leads patients to self-medicate with other opioid-like drugs to alleviate their discomfort; this of course leads to a continuation of the addiction.

Clonidine & opioid withdrawal

A general increase in CNS activity is seen during withdrawal from opioids, nicotine, and alcohol. This increase is thought to be due to the action of NE. Clonidine/Catapres (used to treat hypertension) can be helpful in lessening these symptoms. Clonidine stimulates alpha-adrenoreceptors in the brain stem. This action results in reduced sympathetic outflow from the central nervous system which leads to a decrease in the agitation that usually occurs during withdrawal.

Clonidine is administered either by transdermal skin patch or sublingually (under the tongue). It does not have to pass through the gastrointestinal tract; a major advantage considering the GI disturbances which are frequently present during opioid withdrawal. The usual clonidine regimen for heroin detoxification takes seven days (Fingerhood, et al., 2001).

Adverse effects of clonidine

People complain of tiredness and *dysphoria* (feeling bad) during clonidine treatment (Fingerhood, et al., 2001). This most likely is due to a combination of opioid withdrawal symptoms and to the clonidine.

Naltrexone for opioid withdrawal

Naltrexone/Revia/Vivitrol is a mixed narcotic antagonist and agonist. Taken orally, it is useful for people who have already been detoxified, and it has been found helpful in preventing relapse. Due to its strong affinity for opioid receptors, a person taking naltrexone will not get "high" if opioids are used because the opioid cannot displace the naltrexone at the receptor. Administration of naltrexone will cause withdrawal in someone who is currently addicted to opioids. Agonist (opioid-like) effects are minimal. Taking naltrexone after detox leads to increased production of endorphins which leads to feelings of well-being (Rabinowitz, et al., 2002).

Methadone withdrawal & methadone maintenance

Opioid addicts can receive methadone either as a way to gradually withdraw from opioid use, or as a way to continue using (the methadone) while remaining free from the criminal activity involved in obtaining drugs illegally. The risks to addicts associated with illegal drugs, such as infection with HIV or hepatitis C through contaminated needles, are a major public health concern.

Methadone is usually given in an oral form and dispensed daily through licensed methadone clinics. Methadone is an opioid and causes physical dependency. There will be withdrawal symptoms if a person on methadone decides to decrease the dose or stop taking the drug (Chiang & Goldfrank, 1990).

Buprenorphine & opioid withdrawal

Two sublingual formulations are now available to aid in withdrawal for those who are opioid dependent. The drug buprenorphine/Subutex is intended for the initial stages of withdrawal, and buprenorphine+naloxone/Suboxone is used during the

Time-line for Opioid Withdrawal

6 – 12 HOURS	18 – 24 HOURS	24 – 36 hours
Initial symptoms are:	• NAUSEA	• DIARRHEA
• YAWNING	• VOMITING	• DEHYDRATION
• RUNNY EYES	• HIGHER BLOOD PRESSURE	**48 – 72 hours**
• ANXIETY	• FASTER PULSE RATE	• SYMPTOMS PEAK AND BEGIN TO LESSEN
Followed by:	• FASTER RESPIRATORY RATE	**7 – 10 days**
• HOT & COLD FLASHES	• INCREASED BODY TEMPERATURE	• SYMPTOMS GRADUALLY DISAPPEAR
• APPETITE LOSS		
• MUSCLE CRAMPS		
• INSOMNIA		Table 8.2

maintenance phase of treatment. Buprenorphine blocks most of the effects of heroin, which both discourages relapse and safeguards against overdose. Buprenorphine causes less sedation and dysphoria than methadone. A patient who is taking buprenorphine+naloxone will be unable to get high if opioids are taken. The main advantage of these newer compounds is that they are available for patients to take home, eliminating the need to visit a clinic every day, as is required with methadone treatment. Some adverse effects are:

- sweating
- nausea
- sleep difficulties
- mood swings
- headaches and flu-like symptoms (Benson, 2003)

Rapid detox

Rapid detox is a newer and somewhat controversial drug-detoxification method. It is primarily being used for people addicted to opioids. The treatment can take place over a long weekend and costs over $10,000. The rapid-detox centers claim to have success rates as high as 60% (these claims have not been independently validated) compared to the 15% to 30% success rates for opioid addicts who complete traditional treatment.

A full medical work-up is required before the procedure. The treatment usually takes place in a hospital Intensive Care Unit (ICU) and is overseen by an anesthesiologist with a team of nurses and technicians. The patient is put under general anesthesia and then naloxone is administered. Because the patient is asleep, there is no conscious experience of the unpleasant symptoms that occur during the initial phase of opioid withdrawal. When the anesthesia wears off the patient is given medication to sleep and goes home the next morning. After treatment, the patient either takes naltrexone once a day for up to nine months, or has a naltrexone pellet implanted every six weeks. If the person does use opioids after the detox treatment, the naltrexone will prevent the experience of getting high. Post-treatment counseling is also usually provided (Simon, 2002).

Other Treatments for Severe Pain

Ziconotide, a new drug for pain

Ziconotide/Prialt is a synthetic form of a compound found in a mollusk, the cone snail. It is approved for the treatment of severe, chronic pain that does not respond to other pain medications. It is one of a new type of painkillers called N-type calcium channel blockers. Ziconotide is 1000 times more potent than morphine. It is delivered into the spinal cord through a pump implanted in the abdomen (Prommer, 2006; Wang, et al., 2000). The most frequent side effects are nausea and dizziness. This drug is not an opioid and does not interact with the opioid receptors.

ANALGESIC IMPLANTS

Implants allow people with severe pain to receive medication at a constant rate and without interruption. With this method pain medications are usually more effective, lower doses can be used if the medication is taken before the pain becomes severe, and as a result the adverse effects are lessened. Using implants is also very convenient and avoids the risk of overdose (Prommer, 2006). The adverse effects of opioids still occur but are decreased due to the lower dose required to control the pain.

NICOTINE ANALOGS

It has been known since the 1930s that nicotine, though not an opioid, is helpful for relieving pain. Because of its addictive and toxic effects, it is not used routinely in combination with other analgesics. Researchers are exploring nicotine analogs that are analgesic but do not have the adverse effects caused by opioids (Flood & Daniel, 2004).

DORSAL ROOT SURGERY

Pain messages are carried from the pelvic organs through a section of spinal cord known as the dorsal column. Cutting this tiny nerve bundle stops most pelvic pain messages from reaching the brain. It is not known yet whether cutting this pathway will deprive the patient of other important functions, or eliminate useful pain messages that might alert the CNS of a medical problem. Effects of the surgery are often temporary, and pain may return and be even more severe than before. Even with these potential limitations, the surgery is useful for patients in severe pain (Chen & Tu, 2006; Simpson, 1999).

NERVE-CELL-DESTROYING TOXINS

Methods are being developed to destroy the nerve cells that transmit chronic-pain messages to the brain. This is done by attaching a toxin to a neurotransmitter known to be involved in pain transmission called Substance P. The Substance P will carry the toxin to the cells which are transmitting the pain signal. Compounds are being tested on animals to see if this method works, and a drug is being sought that would temporarily disrupt the pain signal, but not kill the nerve cells, so that the process would be reversible. The main risk of this method is that protective sensations, in addition to those of chronic pain, could be lost when nerve cells are treated in this way (Wiley & Kline, 2000; Wiley & Lappi, 2003).

Direct Relevance to Psychotherapy

The presence of chronic and severe pain, although in itself not life-threatening, leads many people to feelings of helplessness, physical dependence, and frequently to suicidal thoughts and actions. The search continues for compounds to treat severe and chronic pain that do not cause physical dependence or have other serious adverse effects.

Health-care providers are beginning to recognize that one way of helping patients with chronic pain is through understanding their personality characteristics. Using the strengths of an individual's personality as an asset can facilitate the treatment of their pain (Gatchel & Weisberg, 2000).

Pain medications can reduce a client's access to unconscious or disturbing material, thereby decreasing the effectiveness of psychotherapy. The degree to which therapy is influenced depends upon the client's dose and level of tolerance to the specific drug.

Since pain medications are often addictive, it is important to be aware that clients may be currently addicted, in withdrawal, or in recovery from an addiction. All of these conditions will affect psychotherapy, as will severe pain. Psychotherapists are frequently called upon for support and wisdom by clients who are in physical as well as emotional pain, others who are addicted to pain killers, and some who are looking for alternative methods for dealing with their pain.

The best way to be of assistance is to be aware of the options available, including psychiatric evaluation when indicated. It is important to discuss all the available options with the client in order to help the client determine which specific course of action is likely to be most effective.

References for Chapter 8

Ansari, A. (2000). The efficacy of newer antidepressants in the treatment of chronic pain: A review of the current literature. *Harv. Rev. Psychiatry*, 7, 257–277.

Avellanosa, A. & West, C. (1982). Experience with transcutaneous electrical nerve stimulation for relief of intractable pain in cancer patients. *J. Med.*, 13(3), 203–213.

Benson, E. (2003). A new treatment for addiction. *Monitor on Psychology*, June, 18–20.

Chen, H. & Tu, Y. (2006). *Advances in Functional and Repairative Neurosurgery* (Part 3). Springer: Vienna. 73-75.

Chiang, W. & Goldfrank, L. (1990). Substance withdrawal. *Emergency Medicine Clinics of North America*, 8(3), 613–631.

Drake, S. & Xador, D. (1996). Fatal heroin 'overdose': A review. *Addiction*, 91, 1765-672.

Fingerhood, M., Thompson, M. & Jasinski, D. (2001). A comparison of clonidine and buprenorphine in the outpatient treatment of opiate withdrawal. *Substance Abuse*, 22(3), 193–199.

Flood, P. & Daniel, D. (2004). Intranasal nicotine for post-operative pain treatment. *Anesthesiology*, 101(6), 1417-421.

Gatchel, R. & Weisberg, J. (2000). *Personality Characteristics of Patients with Pain*. Washington, D.C.: American Psychological Association.

Gol, A. (1967). Relief of pain by electrical stimulation of the septal area. *J. Neurol. Sci.*, 5(1), 115–120.

Griffin, K. (2005). Beat pain step by step: With all the new warnings which drug is safest for you? *AARP*, July & August, 30, 81.

Joranson, D., Cleeland, C., Weissman, D. & Gilson, A. (1992). Opioids for chronic cancer and non-cancer pain: A survey of state medical board members. Retrieved October 12, 2003, from http://www.ampainsoc.org/

Lazorthes, Y., Verdie, J., Bastide, R., Lavados, A. & Descouens, D. (1985). Spinal versus intraventricular chronic opiate administration with implantable drug delivery devices for cancer pain. *Appl. Neurophysiol.*, 48(1–6), 234–241.

Leo, R. (2002). *A Concise Guide to Pain Management for Psychiatrists.* Washington, DC.: American Psychiatric Press.

Mantyh, P. (2000). Understanding substance P and the substance P receptor. Presented at the XXIInd Congress of the Collegium Internationale Neuro-Psychopharmacologicum (CINP); July 10, 2000; Brussels, Belgium. Abstract.

National Centers for Health Statistics. (2006). *Chartbook on Trends in the Health of Americans.* Special Feature: Pain. Retrieved March 20, 2010: http://www.cdc.gov/nchs/data/hus/hus06.pdf.

Prommer, E. (2006). Ziconotide: A new option for refractory pain. *Drugs Today,* 42(6), 369.

Rabinowitz, J., Cohen, H. & Atias, S. (2002). Outcomes of naltrexone maintenance following ultrarapid opiate detoxification versus intensive inpatient detoxification. *Am. J. Addict.*, 11(1), 52–56.

Schlegel, S. (1987). General characteristics of nonsteroidal anti-inflammatory drugs. In: Paulus, H. E., Furst, D. E. & Dromgoole, S. H. (Eds.) *Anti-inflammatory agents, Nonsteroidal. Vol. 16. Drugs for Rheumatic Disease.* New York: Churchill Livingstone. 203–226.

Simon, D. (2002). Rapid opioid detoxification using opioid antagonists: History, theory and the state of the art. *Perspect. Psychiatr. Care,* 36(4), 113–120.

Simpson, S. (1999). Pain, pain, go away: Snipping a nerve pathway in the spinal cord may bring instant relief. *Science News*, 155, 108–110.

Ventafridda, V., Bianchi, M., Ripamonti, C., Sacerdote, P., De Conno, F., Zecca, E. & Panerai, A. (1990). Studies on the effects of antidepressant drugs on the antinociceptive action of morphine and on plasma morphine in rat and man. *Pain*, 43(2), 155–162.

Wang, Y., Pettus, M., Gao, D., Phillips, C. & Bowersox, S. (2000). Effects of intrathecal administration of ziconotide, a selective neuronal N-type calcium channel blocker, on mechanical allodynia and heat hyperalgesia in a rat model of postoperative pain. *Pain*, 84(2), 151-158.

Wiley, R. & Kline, I. (2000). Neuronal lesioning with axonally transported toxins. *J. Neurosci. Methods,* 103(1), 73–82.

Wiley, R. & Lappi, D. (2003). Targeted toxins in pain. *Adv. Drug Delivery Reviews*, 55(8), 1043-054.

Chapter 9

Consciousness-Altering Drugs

Our normal waking consciousness, rational consciousness as we call it, is but one special type of consciousness, wilst all about it, parted from it by the filmiest of screens, there lie potential forms of consciousness entirely different....No account of the universe in its totality can be final which leaves these other forms of consciousness quite disregarded.

William James

Over the years this group of drugs has been referred to by many different names, including psycholytic, psychotomimetic, empathogenic, and entheogenic, to mention just a few. In 1956, LSD researcher Humphrey Osmond (Hoffer & Osmond, 1967) coined the term "psychedelic" (mind-revealing) by combining the Greek roots *psyche* (mind or soul) and *delos* (revealing or manifesting).

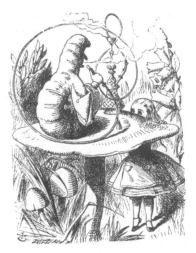

There is no one term or phrase that adequately describes the different qualities and effects of the drugs included in this category. The one quality they all share is the ability to dramatically alter consciousness and to change one's experience of reality. These drugs can affect perception, emotions, cognition, and various combinations of these experiences. There is a high degree of unpredictability of response with some of these drugs. Different people's responses to the same drug may vary, and one person's response to the same drug, taken at different times, may also vary.

Set, setting, drug

This class of drugs is unique in that the nature and intensity of each person's experience is greatly influenced by the set and setting in which the drug is taken. "Set" refers to internal mind set. One's expectations, fears, and previous experiences all influence one's set. "Setting" refers to the external setting in which the drug is taken. The experience will be very different if a drug is taken at a rock concert, in one's home, in a sunny meadow, or in any environment with special significance (Leary, et al., 1963). As the connections between the mind and body are better understood, it is becoming more widely accepted that responses to many drugs, not only those in this category, are influenced by set and setting. This influence is so great with psychedelics that, if they are used, a person must consciously design the set and setting in a way that facilitates the goal for the experience.

Marijuana & Hashish

Marijuana, which refers to the dried leaves and flowering tops of the plants *Cannabis sativa* (C. sativa) and *Cannabis indica* (C. indica), is known by many names. Some examples are pot, weed, reefer, grass, and bhang. Hashish, often called "hash," is made from the resin that forms at the plant's flowering tips.

Cannabis has a long history as a medicinal plant and has been used in many cultures for treating a variety of ailments. In the United States, the widespread use of cannabis compounds for medical purposes is well-documented. It was a standard entry in the *U.S. Pharmacopoeia* (*USP*) until it was removed from the 1942 edition after the criminalization of its use in 1937 (Whitebread, 1995). There has been renewed interest in its medicinal uses since about 1971, and the controversy over its value as a medicine, and its danger as a drug of abuse, continues to rage in America. Many states have decriminalized it for medical use, but under the Controlled Substances Act of 1970, the Department of Justice defines it as a Schedule I drug, a narcotic with a high potential for abuse and no accepted medical value (the same classification as heroin). Despite government assertions, many doctors believe it does have medical uses and is especially effective for:

- improving appetite   • decreasing pain
- reducing intraocular pressure of glaucoma
- relieving nausea resulting from chemotherapy
- decreasing nausea from medications used to treat HIV (Zimmer & Morgan, 1997).

There is evidence that marijuana can be used as part of treatment for alcohol, heroin, and amphetamine dependence (Krupitsky, et al., 2002; McClusky, 1997). In 2008, 25.8 million Americans age 12 and older had used marijuana at least once in the year prior to being surveyed (National Institute on Drug Abuse {NIDA}, 2008).

Marijuana is unique in that it has stimulant, sedative, and hallucinogenic effects. The specific type of effect one gets is strongly influenced by the dose. Cannabis contains over 400 compounds, many of which are psychoactive. The main psychoactive compound is delta-9-tetrahydrocannabinol (THC).

Route of administration

The most common route of administration in the U.S. is via the lungs by smoking. When marijuana is smoked, the blood in the lungs absorbs the THC and quickly transports it to the brain. The peak of intensity occurs soon after inhalation. Marijuana can also be absorbed through the GI tract when eaten (usually in cookies or brownies). Absorption is much slower than when smoked, and the effects may continue to increase for two to three hours after ingestion. Due to the slow rate of absorption it is much more difficult to control the dose with ingestion. If marijuana is smoked, most symptoms usually fade after a few hours; if eaten, symptoms last longer (Selden, et. al., 1990).

Metabolism

Marijuana is metabolized primarily by the liver. Because THC is fat-soluble, it is excreted very slowly. One week after ingestion, 25% to 30% of the THC consumed remains in the body. Traces of marijuana may be detectable for as long as 30 days after ingestion (Selden, et. al., 1990).

PHYSICAL & COGNITIVE EFFECTS OF MARIJUANA INTOXICATION

The common symptoms of marijuana intoxication are:

- a state of euphoria
- sense of time slowing down
- enhanced sensitivity to humor
- feeling remote and withdrawn
- feelings of relaxation
- alienation
- feelings of paranoia
- difficulty concentrating
- short-term impairment of memory (Hall, 1995; Selden, et al., 1990; Zimmer & Morgan, 1997).

Physiological changes–acute

The acute effect of THC on the respiratory system is one of bronchodilation (opening of bronchial tubes). There is a dose-dependent decrease in cognitive and psychomotor performance. At higher doses, driving can be impaired (Hall, 1995; Selden, et al., 1990; Zimmer & Morgan, 1997).

THC also causes:

- an increase in heart rate
- increased appetite
- lower skin temperature
- decreased intraocular pressure
- red eyes
- decreased salivation

Physiological changes–long-term

Alteration of sleep architecture is seen with marijuana use. REM sleep decreases, Stage 4 sleep increases, and total sleep time increases (Hall, 1995; Selden, et al., 1990; Zimmer & Morgan, 1997).

Tolerance

Tolerance to the effects of cannabis develops with daily use. A mild physical dependence also develops. People often smoke cannabis to decrease anxiety; over time, higher doses are needed to obtain this effect (Selden, et. al., 1990).

Withdrawal

Symptoms of cannabis withdrawal are the opposite of those that occur with intoxication. Some of these are:

- restlessness
- anorexia
- vomiting
- tremors
- irritability
- disturbed sleep
- nausea
- diarrhea

Most of these symptoms are seen when any drug with a sedating effect is stopped after someone has become habituated to it. Interestingly, some people who have smoked marijuana daily for years do not feel that they are physically dependent. Men are more likely than women to become dependent, and adolescents are at greater risk than adults (Selden, et al., 1990).

Antimotivational syndrome

This syndrome defines a pattern of changes that has been noted in some daily users. Symptoms reflect a decrease in the anxiety necessary to get things done. Frequently seen are a general loss of motivation, apathy, and a lack of concern for the future.

Some of the symptoms may persist long after the drug's initial intoxicating effects have worn off. These include a loss of ambition, impaired memory, a loss of effectiveness, difficulty concentrating, and a diminished ability to carry out long-term plans. These symptoms often lead to a decline in work or school performance. It usually takes several weeks after the marijuana use is stopped before the syndrome disappears completely (Selden, et al., 1990). This may be due to the slow release of the THC stored in fat cells.

There is controversy over whether marijuana is the cause of this syndrome, or whether marijuana is used as a way of self-medicating to alleviate symptoms of depression. It is not known whether the antimotivational syndrome is reflecting symptoms of an underlying depression or if the lack of motivation is being caused by the daily use of marijuana.

Effects of marijuana on the respiratory system

With long-term use, inflammatory changes take place in the lung tissue which can cause obstructive pulmonary disease, and eventually lead to a decrease in one's ability to get air into the lungs (bronchoconstriction). Anyone with a breathing disorder (e.g., asthma, bronchitis, emphysema) who smokes marijuana will experience a worsening of the disorder over time (Selden, et al., 1990; Hall, 1995).

The U.S. government prohibits the possession of marijuana. Since there are no regulations insuring its safe cultivation, marijuana obtained "on the street" may contain unknown contaminants and pesticides. In contrast to a cigarette, a marijuana "joint" is usually smoked down very far or consumed completely, leading to ingestion of more of the tars. It has not been determined whether smoking marijuana increases or decreases the risk for lung cancer (Guzman, 2003; Kogan, 2005; Munson, et al., 1975).

Effects of marijuana on sexual functioning

Marijuana can affect sexual functioning in various ways. Some claim that marijuana has aphrodisiac qualities and causes an enhancement of the sexual experience. This may be due to a decrease in anxiety, an increased enhancement of the senses, or both. Studies show that smoking marijuana causes a suppression of testicular function, and may also suppress ovarian function. These effects are relevant for anyone who wants to conceive a child and for anyone with known fertility problems (Hall, 1995).

Other effects of marijuana

Women of childbearing age need to be made aware that during pregnancy the THC molecule crosses the placental barrier and passes into the bloodstream of the fetus. THC is also found in the breast milk of nursing mothers.

Studies have shown that marijuana may be harmful to patients who are immunocompromised. This is of particular concern for HIV patients or anyone who has an autoimmune disease (Hall, 1995). The

potentially harmful compounds include:
- cannabinoids • pyrolyzed gasses • particulate matter
- contaminants (adulterants, pesticides, various
  fungi and their metabolites)(Hall, 1995)

Marijuana and psychosis

The research on the link between psychosis and smoking marijuana remains equivocal. A review of the literature (Moore, et al., 2007) indicates a range of increased risk of a psychotic illness for marijuana users from 50% to 200%, with the average being about 100% (double the risk of a matched population who do not use marijuana). The risk appeared to increase with dose. Other researchers disagree with these findings, pointing out that while marijuana use has fluctuated since the 1940s, when records of use began, through its peak in 1979, the rate of people diagnosed with schizophrenia has remained flat or may have declined (Fergusson, 2004).

Experts do agree, that for people at high risk for psychosis (e.g., those who have a family history of this disorder), marijuana use is correlated with a first psychotic episode at an earlier age than for those who do not use the drug (Henquet, et al., 2005).

Possible medical uses for marijuana

In the last few years, after an almost 40 year ban, researchers have been able to obtain marijuana for experimental purposes. Although it is still too early to be certain of the final outcomes of the studies, some interesting findings, and potential medical uses, have already come to light. For a complete update on current research on many psychedelic drugs see www.maps.org.

Cannabinoids and pain

In a study using rats, it was found that marijuana-like compounds found in the brain (cannabinoids) rose rapidly after an injury. In this phenomena, called stress-induced analgesia, it is believed that the cannabinoids are released in order to decrease the pain (Hohmann, et al., 2005).

Medical marijuana

Sativex is a medication developed to treat multiple sclerosis (Wade, et al., 2006) and the severe pain caused by nerve damage. It is sprayed under the tongue and absorbed through the mucus membranes. Sativex includes all of the components of the cannabis plant whereas Marinol, the other medicinal compound from marijuana, is synthetic and contains only THC. The manufacturer claims that Sativex does not cause the intoxication that people usually experience when smoking marijuana. Sativex was approved for medicinal use in Canada in 2005.

Cannabinoids and cancer suppression

In 1975 it was discovered (Munson et al.) that cannabinoids suppress lung carcinoma cell growth. The mechanism of this action was shown to be inhibition of DNA synthesis. Antiproliferative action on some other cancer cells was also found (De Petrocellis, et al., 1998). A few years ago, almost simultaneously, two groups resumed research on the antiproliferative effects of cannabinoids on cancer cells: De Petrocellis et. al., (1998) found that cannabinoids inhibit breast cancer-cell-proliferation, and Guzman's (2003) group found that cannabinoids inhibit the growth of glioma cells. Today, a wide array of cancer cell lines that are affected in this way are known, and some of the mechanisms involved have been elucidated (Kogan, 2005).

Cannabinoids and neurogenesis

Experiments seem to indicate that the endogenous cannabinoids promote the growth and generation of new nerve cells in the rat hippocampus. The generation of new nerves is thought to be a possible mechanism for the anxiety reduction properties of marijuana (Jiang, et al., 2005).

Cannabinoids as antibiotics

There is evidence (Appendino, et al., 2008) that Cannabis sativa contains cannabinoids with the potential to treat antibiotic resistant infections. These cannabinoids show potent activity against a variety of methicillin-resistant Staphylococcus aureus (MRSA) strains.

Cannabinoid antagonist for smoking cessation

The selective CB1 cannabinoid antagonist rimonabant (SR141716) decreases the craving for nicotine and enables longer abstinence from smoking (Cohen, et al., 2005). The Phase III clinical trial of this drug (for effectiveness and safety) has been completed (Efficacy and Safety of Rimonabant, 2009). There is some evidence that the use of rimonabant prevents the weight gain usually associated with smoking cessation. The complete results of this trial were not yet published at the time of this writing.

Psychological treatment for marijuana users

Many modalities of therapy have been tried with habitual users of marijuana who express a desire to stop. These include family therapy, cognitive-behavioral and motivational treatments, community reinforcement programs, and therapy supplemented with discussions of family dynamics. All the treatment strategies are equally successful. One year after completion, all modalities of treatment show success rates about 30% better than control groups receiving no treatment (Selden, et al., 1990).

Lysergic Acid Diethylamide (LSD, "acid")

History of LSD

Ergot-like compounds may have been derived from grain infected with a fungus called "wheat rust" which develops on wheat and rye. This naturally-occurring fungus contains ergot compounds which dilate blood vessels, which in high doses can result in bleeding disorders. Ingesting infected grain causes a potentially fatal disease known as *St. Anthony's Fire*. The symptoms are burning sensations in the hands and feet and hallucinations. High doses of ergot can lead to extensive internal bleeding.

There are hints that a compound like LSD was part of the annual rituals known as the Eleusinian Mysteries which were practiced in ancient Greece for 2,000 years. The participants were not allowed to talk about what went on in the rituals, hence "mysteries." Pottery has survived from this period which is decorated with paintings of the goddess of the harvest, Demeter, holding sheaves of wheat. This supports the idea that wheat infected with an ergot compound was used in the rites. What took place at Eleusis is not known, and experts differ as to what specific compound, if any, was involved in the rites (Wasson, et al., 1988).

In 1943, Dr. Albert Hofmann, while working as a research chemist at Sandoz Pharmaceutical Laboratories in Switzerland, was searching for a compound to act as a "blood stimulant." He was using ergot derivatives because of their known action on blood vessels. He would sometimes try compounds on himself, as scientists occasionally do. Most drugs are active at doses ranging from one milligram to hundreds of milligrams, so when he took a mere 250 *micrograms* of LSD (0.25 mg) he believed it was a minute dose (as it would be for almost any other drug). Hofmann soon discovered that 250 micrograms of LSD caused a potent and long-lasting change in his perceptual and emotional state (Hofmann, 1980).

LSD is effective in doses as low as 50 micrograms (.05 mg), and its effects (popularly called a "trip") last 12 to 16 hours after a single dose. It may be that a metabolite of LSD, and not the LSD itself, causes the changes in perception and feelings. Another theory is that taking LSD may lead to a cascade of events in the CNS which then leads to its effects. Estimates are that 13.2 million Americans over age 12 have tried LSD at least once (up from 8.1 million in 1985) (NIDA, 2001; U.S. Dept. of Justice, 1993).

Effects of LSD

The LSD experience varies greatly from person to person. Factors of set, setting, and the amount of the drug taken, all influence the experience. Frequently, there is an alteration of perception and feeling which can range in intensity from very mild to extreme. Depending on many factors, the experience may also vary from wildly ecstatic to utterly hellish. Many of the variables that can influence expectations, such as personal history, state of mind, and reports by friends, are difficult to quantify.

Tolerance to LSD

With daily use, tolerance to LSD will develop in two to four days. Although some psychological dependence may develop, there are no signs of physical dependence with long-term or repeated use. Cross-tolerance develops between LSD, mescaline, and psilocybin (Hofmann, 1980). These compounds have different chemical structures, but all have similar psychedelic effects. The cross-tolerance hints that there may be a common final site of action for these drugs.

Toxic reaction to LSD

There are no adverse physical effects due to ingesting even very large amounts of LSD, although there have been many reports of extremely upsetting and dangerous psychological experiences. Intensity of experience is related to size of dose, but there is no direct relationship between the dose and whether the experience will be pleasant or terrifying. Taking LSD may uncover unconscious fears or fantasies that may be undesirable and frightening. The unpleasant symptoms most frequently reported are paranoia, frightening delusions, and agitation (NIDA, 2001).

People with a mood disorder or schizophrenia may become mentally disorganized after taking LSD, and their symptoms may not clear when the LSD has worn off. In cases where symptoms continue long afterward, diagnosis and treatment for the underlying disorder is appropriate (NIDA, 2001).

Antianxiety drugs (BzRAs in particular) can be given to decrease agitation. Some people report that taking large doses of vitamins B and C also can be helpful in counteracting the effects of LSD. All of the drug's effects usually are gone within 24 hours and the pre-drug state of consciousness is usually regained.

LSD psychotherapy

The use of LSD as an aid to psychotherapy has been studied extensively by Stan Grof and his colleagues and is explored in detail in his book, *LSD Psychotherapy* (1980). The researchers found that using LSD as an adjunct to psychotherapy lessened defenses and allowed access to affective experiences and memories that had previously not been available to the conscious mind. They believed that this facilitated the process of psychotherapy.

Prior to its criminalization, LSD was also used experimentally to create what was called a "functional psychosis." This state mimicked a psychotic state but was drug-induced and time-limited. It was hoped that the ability to create a psychotic state under experimental conditions would increase understanding and yield information that could be used in developing new treatment methods. Due to legal restrictions, research was discontinued in the U.S. after 1966.

Dimethyltryptamine (DMT)

DMT occurs naturally in some South American plants and is used in shamanic practices throughout the Amazon basin. The usual forms of administration are via the nasal membranes by snorting, through the lungs by smoking, and by sprinkling the compounds onto marijuana and then smoking. DMT is destroyed by stomach acid so it is not effective when taken by mouth.

All of these methods cause an immediate onset of effects. The DMT experience usually lasts for about 30 minutes, after which the user returns to a normal state. DMT is sometimes said to have effects like short-acting LSD. It causes vivid visual hallucinations and sometimes a loss of awareness of one's surroundings (Metzner, 1999). It can be described as going to the peak of an intense LSD experience in the time it takes to inhale. This is likely to be extremely disorienting and frightening for anyone who is not both very familiar and very comfortable with the LSD experience.

Phenylethylamines

All phenylethylamines are structurally similar to dopamine, norepinephrine, and the amphetamines. Some examples are:

- methylenedioxyamphetamine (MDA)
- methylenedioxymethamphetamine (MDMA, "ecstasy," "X")
- 3-methoxy-4,5-methylenedioxyphenylisopropylamine (MMDA)
- 3,4,5-trimethoxyphenethylamine (mescaline/peyote)

It is said that MDA and similar drugs can be synthesized from safrol and myristicin, two oils derived from nutmeg. Nutmeg is referred to as a narcotic fruit in the *Atharva Veda*, one of a small number of ancient Indian texts that deals with healing and prolonging life.

Before 1985, it was not illegal to use phenylethylamines to facilitate psychotherapy. In *The Healing Journey* (1974), Claudio Naranjo wrote about the use of MDA and MMDA in conjunction with psychotherapy. He calls these drugs "feeling enhancers." They are also called "empathogens," a designation for drugs that enhance empathy. When his patients were under the influence of one of these compounds, Naranjo observed an intensification of feeling, access to underlying experiences, and spontaneous age-regression.

METHYLENEDIOXYMETHAMPHETAMINE (MDMA)

MDMA ("ecstasy") has become popular as a "club drug" at dance events known as "raves." MDMA is believed to induce feelings of love, decrease fear (Teter & Guthrie, 2001), and facilitate the "working through" of psychological material by reducing defenses. Before it became illegal, many psychotherapists were using MDMA to facilitate psychotherapy (Adamson, 1984; Greer & Tolbert 1998).

MDMA causes the release of all stored serotonin from the vesicles of the nerve cell. After release the reuptake of 5-HT is blocked (Solowij, 1993). Neurodegeneration is seen in animal studies. The long-term effects of MDMA on human brain cells is still under investigation (Fleckenstein et al., 2007).

Mushrooms, Peyote, Ayahuasca & Ibogaine

PSILOCYBIN MUSHROOMS

Stropharia cubensis is the mushroom most frequently used to attain an altered state of awareness during shamanic rituals by Native Americans in the U.S. and Mexico. The mushrooms, which usually grow on the dung of deer or cattle, are used in religious ceremonies for divination, and by shamans in healing ceremonies. Considered sacred for 3,000 years, they are depicted in stone sculptures found in Guatemala dating from around 1000 BCE.

The main active ingredient is psilocybin (4-phosphoryloxy-N, N-dimethyltryptamine); an accompanying compound, psilocin (4-hydroxyl-N, N-dimethyltryptamine) is also present in much smaller amounts. Psilocybin, which is in the chemical group called indolealkylamines, is similar in molecular structure to serotonin (Wasson, 1980).

Effects of psilocybin

The Aztecs used psilocybin in rituals with the belief that while under the effects of these mushrooms they could cure the sick, talk to the gods, and talk to the deceased. Ingesting these mushrooms causes fundamental alterations in consciousness, including changes in the perception of time, space, and in both the psychic and bodily selves. The sense of being an objective observer of oneself (being on the outside looking in) is sometimes experienced. This experience of objectivity can lead to insights into one's motives and behaviors that are not accessible during ordinary consciousness.

Sight and hearing are greatly enhanced; this may be experienced as exaggerations in perception, or as auditory and visual hallucinations. Also enhanced is the ability to clearly recall long-forgotten events, often from early childhood (Wasson, 1980). For this reason psilocybin may also prove to be useful in facilitating psychotherapy.

Psilocybin for OCD

A recent study (2006) done by Dr. Francisco Moreno's group using psilocybin to treat patients with Obsessive Compulsive Disorder demonstrated the safety of psilocybin in a controlled setting and also showed positive results. A significant decrease of OCD symptoms occurred in all nine patients. Most of the patients symptoms came back gradually after 24 to 72 hours, although one patient had a remission of symptoms for six months.

The conclusion of the experiment was that, in a controlled clinical environment, psilocybin was safe to use in subjects with OCD and was associated with acute reductions in core OCD symptoms in several subjects (Moreno, et al., 2006). Currently, there is no treatment that eases symptoms of this disorder as rapidly as psilocybin.

Psilocybin for cluster headaches

The authors (Sewell, et al., 2006) interviewed 53 cluster headache patients who had used psilocybin or lysergic acid diethylamide (LSD) to treat their headaches. Twenty-two of 26 psilocybin users reported that psilocybin aborted their attacks; 25 of 48 psilocybin users and seven of eight LSD users reported cluster-period termination (cluster headaches usually occur in a series); 18 of 19 psilocybin users and four of five LSD users reported longer headache-free periods of remission. Further research on the effects of psilocybin and LSD on cluster headache seems appropriate.

FLY AGARIC MUSHROOM

The fly agaric mushroom (*Amanita muscarina*) is native to Lapland, Siberia, and other regions in extreme northern latitudes and is used by the Sami and Siberian shamans in their healing practices. The active ingredients are muscimole and muscarine. Researcher Gordon Wasson has investigated these mushrooms extensively and believes they are the Soma known by ancient Indo-Europeans as the "mushroom of immortality" (Wasson, 1980).

These mushrooms have consciousness-changing ability whether

eaten raw, cooked, or dried. Because of the way the ingredients are metabolized, the urine of someone or some animal that has ingested the mushrooms is stronger in narcotic and intoxicating properties than the unmetabolized mushrooms. Shamans often drink the urine of an intoxicated person, their own urine, or the urine of a reindeer that had eaten the mushrooms (Wasson, 1980).

Effects of amanita

The effects begin 15 to 20 minutes after ingestion and last for a few hours. First the person sleeps for about two hours. This is not a normal sleep, as one cannot be roused from it. There is an awareness of external sounds and an experience of colored visions. After awakening, people report feelings of elation that last from three to four hours. During this period, people report a capacity for feats of extraordinary physical strength and find this very enjoyable. Shamans believe that the mushrooms will tell anyone who eats them what ails them when they are sick, explain a dream, show them the upper or underground world, and foretell the future (Wasson, 1980).

PEYOTE

The peyote cactus (*Lophophora williamsii*) is native to an area ranging from near the Rio Grande river and extending south between Mexico's eastern and western Sierra Madre mountain ranges to the Tropic of Cancer. Pre-Columbian art, dating from approximately 100 BCE, depicts the peyote cactus. Today, peyote is used in the shamanic practices of the Huichol Indians and is a sacrament of the Native American Church.

Effects of mescaline

The main psychoactive compound in peyote is mescaline (3,4,5-trimethoxyphenethylamine). Peyote is very bitter and difficult to swallow by itself and is usually ingested as a tea, swallowed in capsules, or ground-up and mixed with food. About 45 minutes after ingestion, most people begin to see brilliantly colored images, particularly geometric designs, and "auras," which appear as halos of light around people and objects. There is an enhancement of auditory, olfactory, gustatory, and tactile sensations. There are feelings of weightlessness, as well as the experience of macroscopia (the ability to observe things with the details greatly magnified, such as watching a candle burning, or ice melting). There is an alteration of one's perception of time and space; time seems to move more slowly, and objects appear to change size (Schultes & Hofmann, 1979).

Most people report less cognitive distortion with peyote than with LSD, and because of this there are fewer anxious reactions. This may be related to size of the dose rather than to the specific compound. Peyote is often taken in a religious or spiritual setting. The use of ritual, and having elders present to guide the session, are also factors that decrease fear (Schultes, & Hofmann, 1979).

AYAHUASCA

Ayahuasca is a compound consisting of at least two main plant substances: The *Banisteriopsis caapi* vine, which contains harmaline (an MAO inhibitor), and *Psychotria viridis*, a green, leafy plant which contains the vision-inducing DMT (see above) or other tryptamine. The hallucinogenic extract has a variety of names, including ayahuasca, caapi, natema, pinde, and yajé (Metzner, 1999).

According to folklore, ayahuasca is the "font of all understanding that reveals the origins of all life." In traditional societies ayahuasca was never used recreationally. A period of ritual cleansing of several weeks was required before a person could partake of the experience. A shaman (curandero) is in charge of the ritual. After nightfall, the brew is passed around, the shaman sings of the visions they will see and then the purging begins. Intense vomiting and diarrhea cleanse the body of parasites and emotional blockages (Metzner, 1999). After this come the visions and "out-of-body" experiences. Several Brazilian churches use ayahuasca as a sacrament. These churches now have branches in the U.S. and many other countries.

Effects of harmaline (the MAOI in ayahuasca)

- nausea/vomiting/diarrhea
- general malaise • dizziness
- numbness of the hands, feet, and face
- visions (considered useful in divination)

Unlike some experiences with other psychedelic drugs, neither color enhancement nor distortions of body-image are present with ayahuasca (Metzner, 1999).

Harmaline overdose

In large doses, harmaline causes tremors and clonic (jerking) convulsions. These effects are related to the inhibition of monoamine oxidase. With toxic doses harmaline causes:

- respiratory arrest • fall in body temperature
- a weakening of cardiac muscles which results in a vasodepressant effect

Tabernanthe iboga use in therapy for addictions

In the West African Bwiti religion ibogaine, an extract from the African plant *Tabernanthe iboga*, is used as a sacrament as a way to "visit the ancestors." Ibogaine is an indole alkaloid that is purported to interrupt heroin addiction and eliminate withdrawal (Alper, et al., 1999).

It is estimated that more than 5000 people have taken ibogaine since an addiction treatment clinic was opened in Amsterdam in the mid 1980s. It is thought that there are now 30-40 clinics world-wide. The U.S. Drug Enforcement Agency has listed ibogaine as a Schedule I substance (like LSD, heroin, and marijuana). Ibogaine is legal in most of the world (Vastag, 2005). Systematic research on its effectiveness for treating addictions is on-going (Kroupa & Wells, 2005).

Salvia divinorum

Salvia divinorum is a species of sage. It is a leafy plant indigenous to Mexico that when chewed or smoked causes intense hallucinations and out-of-body experiences. It has been used for decades by Mazatec shamans for divination in religious ceremonies. The effects are quite brief, lasting only a few minutes (Wasson, 1962).

At this point little is known about any potential long-term effects. Research is being done on the possibilities of using salvia to treat depression or bipolar disorder. The ingredient in the plant that causes the hallucinations is called salvinorin A. It is a unique psychedelic in that it does not react with the serotonin receptors in the brain.

Dissociatives (previously called Dissociative Anesthetics)

This group of drugs (phencyclidine, ketamine, and dextromethorphan) are classified as "dissociatives" due to the frequent out-of-body (dissociative) experiences reported by users and because of the numbing of physical sensation (anesthesia) that accompanies intoxication. These drugs have a small depressant effect on respiration and blood pressure, but much less than most other anesthetics (Baldridge & Bessen, 1990); because of this, ketamine is in some ways a safer anesthetic than many others. When dextromethorphan, which is a cough suppressant and not an anesthetic, was added to the drugs in this class, they became known as dissociatives rather than dissociative anesthetics.

Phencyclidine (PCP)

Until the 1980s, the main drug of abuse in this group (the dissociatives) was PCP ("angel dust"). PCP was originally developed in the 1950s as an intravenous surgical anesthetic. It was never approved for human use because of feelings of delirium and agitation that were experienced by test subjects when emerging from the PCP anesthesia. For intoxication, PCP can be taken orally or mixed with marijuana or tobacco and smoked (NIDA, 2001).

Effects of PCP

Depending on the dose taken and the route of administration, PCP can have hallucinogenic, analgesic, stimulant, and/or depressive effects. A behavioral tolerance develops with chronic use. Although there is no development of physical dependence, a psychological dependence can develop. There will be no physical withdrawal symptoms if use is discontinued. Other symptoms, such as loss of memory and depression, may persist for as long as a year after a chronic user stops taking PCP (NIDA, 2001).

The half-life of PCP is only 45 minutes, but due to its fat-solubility traces of the drug may stay in the body up to three days. In low doses, PCP acts as a CNS depressant. Taking less than a 5 milligram dose causes a state similar to alcohol intoxication. With doses in the 5 mg to 10 mg range, PCP may cause *hyperreflexia* (increased muscle tone), and *catalepsy* (cessation of motion and nonresponsiveness to external stimuli, as in catatonic states) (NIDA, 2001).

PCP intoxication can induce psychotic symptoms that may persist long after the drug has been metabolized, sometimes for months. Psychotic symptoms occur most frequently in people who have a history of mental illness. In these cases, it is important to diagnose and treat the underlying mental disorder (usually with antipsychotic medication) (NIDA, 2001).

Treatment for PCP intoxication

People who are under the influence of PCP often appear agitated and violent. For this reason, it is very important to calm the person as much as possible. This is best accomplished by decreasing external stimuli (putting the person in a dark, quiet room). Emergency room personnel sometimes use restraints to prevent these patients from harming themselves or others. A BzRA such as diazepam is often used to decrease the agitation and muscle hypertonicity. Most symptoms of the intoxication will clear in several hours.

PCP overdose

Symptoms of overdose can occur with a dose of 20 mg or more. Overdose may cause a hypertensive crisis, seizures, and a respiratory depression that can lead to a comatose state. This coma can last for several days and can be fatal. The patient must be hospitalized to establish adequate oxygen intake and for treatment of the hypertension. Diazepam or one of the other BzRAs is usually given to decrease the possibility of seizures.

KETAMINE

Ketamine/Ketalar ("K," "vitamin K," "special K") is 2-2-chlorophenyl-2-methylamino-cyclohexanone. It was developed in 1963 as a general anesthetic for use during major surgery and was used widely in the field during the Vietnam war. Ketamine is a unique drug in that it has hypnotic (sleep producing), analgesic (pain relieving) and amnesic (short-term memory loss) effects; no other drug used in clinical practice combines these three features.

Ketamine is most useful for patients who have respiratory conditions that would put them at increased risk if barbiturates or most other types of general anesthesia were used. It is used as an anesthetic by the military in the field (where hospital backup and support are not available) because of the lower risk of respiratory failure. Ketamine is useful with both the pediatric and elderly populations due to large individual metabolic variations in these groups, which makes it more difficult to calculate the safe and correct dose of other anesthetics.

Although ketamine is legal to use as an anesthetic, it is not widely used due to the problems of dealing with what is termed "emergence phenomena" (the altered states of consciousness experienced as the ketamine wears off). If not prepared beforehand for these experiences, patients may become frightened and difficult to manage as they awaken. For this reason, ketamine is rarely used as a general anesthetic with humans. Since it is very safe, it is often used by veterinarians for surgery on animals.

When used as a recreational drug, ketamine can be taken by intramuscular injection, snorted, or smoked. Its usual effects are feelings of disembodiment, feeling part of the cosmic energy field, and having colorful visions. There is usually no significant emotional response, and it generally does not elicit fear. The experience usually lasts about an hour (NIDA, 2001). A tolerance to the physical effects (numbing, inability to walk) caused by this drug will develop with repeated use.

Other uses for Ketamine

- Ketamine is useful for some severe pain syndromes which are not relieved with other medications, such as the pain of post-herpetic neuralgia.
- There is evidence that it may be useful with patients who have terminal illnesses to help them overcome their fear of death (Jansen, 1996).
- Scientists in Russia have been researching the use of ketamine in conjunction with psychotherapy as a treatment for alcohol and heroin addiction. They have found that psychedelic doses of ketamine led to a significant rate of abstinence and reduced the craving for heroin (Krupitsky, et al., 2002).
- Evidence exists that ketamine may be a drug that has a rapid onset for the treatment of depression (Hampton, 2006). As of 2009 the NIMH was still recruiting subjects for a clinical trial of its effectiveness for this use.

DEXTROMETHORPHAN (DXM)

DXM ("robo") is a cough-suppressing ingredient found in many over-the-counter cold and cough preparations such as Coricidin and Robitussin. In very high doses, DXM can induce experiences of dissociation that may last for up to six hours.

Direct Relevance to Psychotherapy

People of all generations regularly use alcohol, and many who grew up in the 1960s and 1970s experimented extensively with psychedelics and marijuana, and more than a few continue to use these drugs and others, either regularly or intermittently. In addition, a significant percentage of the generations of people who are now in their teens, twenties and thirties has taken LSD, MDMA, ketamine, psilocybin, and various other psychedelic compounds.

Many clients will talk about their drug experiences if they do not receive a negative or judgmental reaction from the therapist. Since these drugs are used so widely, particularly by some populations, it is important that psychotherapists have both an openness to, and an understanding of, the use and effects of the various consciousness-altering drugs. As people grow into their teens, twenties, and thirties, it is common that many will experiment with drugs as a part of their explorations of other states of consciousness. Psychotherapists need to be proactive in exploring whether their clients are experimenting with these drugs.

Most clients will be alert for any hint of judgement or condemnation on the part of the therapist. The ability to stay open and curious to a client's experiences will prove to be the most fruitful approach to gleaning information as to the client's experimentation with, or regular use of, these substances. This openness will allow the therapist and the client to explore, in the therapeutic setting, the meaning and purpose of the client's experiences. A knowledgeable therapist will be able to discuss both adverse and possible positive consequences which might result from the use of these substances.

References for Chapter 9

Adamson, S. (1984). *Through the Gateway of the Heart.* San Francisco, CA: Four Trees Publications.

Alper, K., Lotsof, H., Frenken, G., Luciano, D. & Bastiaans, J. (1999). Treatment of acute opioid withdrawal with ibogaine. *American Journal on Addictions,* 8 (3), 234–42.

Appendino, G., Gibbons, S., Giana, A., Pagani, A., Grassi, G., Stavri, M., Smith, E. & Rahman, M. (2008). Antibacterial cannabinoids from Cannabis sativa: A structure-activity study. *Nat. Prod.,* 71 (8), 1427–430.

Baldridge, E. & Bessen, H. (1990). Phencyclidine. *Emergency Medicine Clinics of North America,* 8(3), 541–550.

Cohen, C., Perrault, G., Griebel, G. & Soubrié, P. (2005). Nicotine-associated cues maintain nicotine-seeking behavior in rats several weeks after nicotine withdrawal: Reversal by the cannabinoid (CB1) receptor antagonist, rimonabant (SR141716). *Neuropsychopharm.,* 30, 145-155.

De Petrocellis, L., Melck, D., Palmisano, A., Bisogno, T., Laezza, C., Bifulco, M. & Di Marzo,

V. (1998). The endogenous cannabinoid anandamide inhibits human breast cancer cell proliferation. *Proc. Nat. Acad. Sciences,* 95(14), 8375–380.

Efficacy and Safety of Rimonabant as an Aid to Smoking Cessation With or Without Nicotine Patch. (2009). Retrieved January 14, 2010. http://clinicaltrials.gov/ct2/show/NCT00458718

Fergusson, D. (2004). Cannabis and psychosis: Two kinds of limitations which attach to epidemiological research. *Addiction,* 99(4), 512-513.

Fleckenstein, A., Volz, T., Riddle, E., Gibb, J. &. Hanson, G. (2007). New insights into the mechanism of action of amphetamines. *Annual Review of Pharmacology and Toxicology,* 47, 681-698.

Grof, S. (1980). *LSD Psychotherapy.* Pomona, CA: Hunter House.

Guzman, M. (2003). Cannabinoids: Potential anticancer agents. *Nat. Rev. Cancer,* 3, 745-55.

Hall, W. (1995). *Project on health implications of cannabis use: A comparative appraisal of health and psychological consequences of alcohol, cannabis, nicotine and opiate use, II. The probable effects of cannabis use.* WHO (World Health Organization). Retrieved September 7, 2003 from www.druglibrary.org/shaffer/hemp/general/who-index.htm.

Hampton, T. (2006). Ketamine for depression. *JAMA,* 296, 1458.

Henquet, C., Krabbendam, L., Spauwen, J., Kaplan, C., Lieb, R., Wittchen, H. & van Os, J. (2005). Prospective cohort study of cannabis use, predisposition for psychosis, and psychotic symptoms in young people. *BMJ,* 1, 330(7481),11.

Hoffer, A. & Osmond, H. (1967). *The Hallucinogens.* New York: Academic Press.

Hofmann, A. (1980). *LSD-My Problem Child, Reflections on Sacred Drugs, Mysticism, and Science.* New York: McGraw-Hill.

Hohmann, A., Suplita, R., Bolton, N., Neely, M., Fegley, D., Mangieri, R., Krey, J., Walke, J., Holmes, P., Crystal, J., Duranti, A., Tontini, A., Mor, M., Tarzia, G. & Piomelli, D. (2005). An endocannabinoid mechanism for stress-induced analgesia. *Nature,* 435, 1108-112.

Jansen, K. (1996). Using ketamine to induce the near-death experience: Mechanism of action and therapeutic potential. *Yearbook for Ethnomedicine and the Study of Consciousness* (Jahrbuch fur Ethnomedizin und Bewubtseinsforschung). Issue 4, 55–81. C. Ratsch; J. R. Baker, (Eds.), Berlin: VWB.

Jiang, W., Zhang, Y., Xiao, L., Van Cleemput, J., Ji, S-P., Bai, G. & Zhang, X. (2005). Cannabinoids promote embryonic and adult hippocampus neurogenesis and produce anxiolytic and antidepressant-like effects. *J. Clin. Invest.,* 115(11), 3104-116.

Kogan, N. (2005). Cannabinoids and Cancer. *Mini Reviews in Medicinal Chemistry,* 5(10), 941-52.

Kroupa, P. & Wells, H. (2005). Ibogaine in the 21st Century. *Multidisciplinary Association for Psychedelic Studies,* XV(1), 21-25.

Krupitsky, E., Burakov, A., Romanova, T., Dunaevsky, I. & Strassman, R. (2002). Ketamine psychotherapy for heroin addiction: Immediate effects and follow-up. *J. Subst. Abuse Treatment,* 23(4), 273–283.

Leary. T., Litwin, G. & Metzner, R. (1963). Reactions to psilocybin administered in a supportive environment. *J. Nervous and Mental Disease,* 137, 561–573.

McClusky, J. (1997). Native American Church peyotism and treatment of alcoholism. *MAPS Bulletin*, VII(4), 3–4.

Metzner, R., (Ed.) (1999). *Ayahuasca: Human Consciousness and the Spirits of Nature.* New York: Thunder's Mouth Press.

Moore, T., Zammit, S., Lingford-Hughes, A., Barnes, T., Jones, P., Burke, M. & Lewis, G. (2007) Cannabis use and risk of psychotic or affective mental health outcomes: A systematic review. *Lancet*, 370(9584), 319-328.

Moreno, F., Wiegand, C., Taitano, E. & Delgado, P. (2006). Safety, tolerability, and efficacy of psilocybin in 9 patients with obsessive-compulsive disorder. *J. Clin. Psychiatry*, 67(11), 1735-740.

Munson, A., Harris, L., Friedman, M., Dewey, W. & Carchman, R. (1975). Antineoplastic activity of cannabinoids. *J. Natl. Cancer Inst.*, 55, 597–602.

Naranjo, C. (1974). *The Healing Journey*. New York: Pantheon Books.

National Institute on Drug Abuse (NIDA), (2008). Retrieved January 14, 2010, http://www.drugabuse.gov/drugpages/marijuana.html

NIDA (2001). Hallucinogens and dissociative drugs: Including LSD, PCP, ketamine, dextromethorphan. *NIH Publication*, Number 01–409.

NIMH (2009). Rapid antidepressant effects of ketamine in major depression. ClinicalTrials.gov Identifier: NCT00088699

Schultes, R. & Hofmann, A. (1979) *Plants of the Gods: Origins of Hallucinogenic Use.* New York: Alfred van der Marck Editions.

Selden, B., Clark, R. & Curry, S. (1990). Marijuana. *Emergency Medicine Clinics of North America*, 8(3), 527–539.

Sewell, R., Halpern, J. & Pope, H. (2006). Response of cluster headache to psilocybin and LSD. *Neurology*, 66(12),1920-922.

Solowij, N. (1993). Ecstasy (3,4-methylenedioxymethamphetamine). *Current Opinion in Psychiatry*, 6, 411–415.

Teter, C. & Guthrie, S. (2001). A comprehensive review of MDMA and GHB: Two common club drugs. *Pharmacotherapy*, 21, 1487–1513.

U.S. Department of Justice, Drug Enforcement Administration. (1993). LSD in the United States.

Vastag, B. (2005). Ibogaine therapy: A vast uncontrolled experiment. *Science*, 308, 345-46.

Wade, D., Makela, P., House, H., Bateman, C. & Robson, P. (2006). Long-term use of a cannabis-based medicine in the treatment of spasticity and other symptoms in multiple sclerosis. *Mult. Scler.*, 12 (5), 639–45.

Wasson, R. (1962). A New Mexican Psychotropic Drug from the Mint Family. *Botanical Museum Leaflets*, Harvard University, 20(3).

Wasson, R., Kramrisch, S., Ott, J. & Ruck, C. (1988). *Persephone's Quest: Entheogens and the Origins of Religion*. New Haven, CT: Yale University Press.

Wasson, R. (1980). *The Wondrous Mushroom*. New York: McGraw-Hill.

Whitebread, C. (1995). The history of the non-medical use of drugs in the United States. A speech to the California Judges Association Annual Conference. Retrieved December 17, 2003 from, http://www.druglibrary.org/schaffer/history/whiteb1.htm

Zimmer, L. & Morgan, J. (1997). *Marijuana Myths, Marijuana Facts: Review of the Scientific Evidence*. New York, NY: The Lindesmith Center.

Chapter 10

Cognition-Enhancing Drugs

The term "nootropic" (acting on the mind) is used to describe a group of drugs which have in common the ability to improve cognition but are chemically unrelated to each other and have diverse pharmacological properties. In the past, when the average life span was only until the mid- 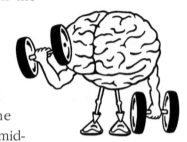 forties, there was little need for cognition-enhancing drugs. But now as the baby-boom generation ages and the World War II generation lives into their nineties and even longer, interest, need, and demand for this group of drugs is rapidly increasing.

The extension of life that comes with modern medicine brings with it an increased need to treat the diseases of the elderly. Of particular concern are the dementias seen in this population. Along with the ever-increasing knowledge of the structural and metabolic changes that take place with aging is the development and testing of new drugs and herbal remedies in the hope of finding more effective treatments for dementia.

Many of these drugs are designed to improve the memory processes of consolidation, retrieval, and learning. Researchers are trying to develop drugs that improve memory and at the same time avoid effects such as insomnia, anorexia, and nervousness which are often experienced with many stimulant drugs.

Alzheimer's Disease

Alzheimer's is a progressive, degenerative disease of the brain which affects one in every eight people aged 65 or older. Currently, this is approximately 5.3 million Americans, three million of whom are living at home and being cared for by family members. The percentage increases to about 50% for people over the age of 85. If no cure is found, the number of people afflicted with Alzheimer's is expected to double by the year 2050 (Alzheimer's Association, 2010).

RISK FACTORS FOR ALZHEIMER'S DISEASE

Heredity and head injury

The two major confirmed risk factors are heredity and head trauma. A moderate concussion in one's medical history doubles the risk of developing Alzheimer's, and a severe concussion more than quadruples the risk.

There are four specific genes now known to increase the risk of Alzheimer's. They are: Apolipoprotein E (APOE), and three additional genes, known as clusterin (APOJ), complement receptor 1 (CR1), and PICALM. These last three have been linked to the typical late-onset form of Alzheimer's (Harold, et al., 2009; Lambert, et al., 2009).

Type 3 diabetes

There is now evidence that the normal brain makes its own insulin. Alzheimer's disease may be caused by what is being called "type 3" diabetes which occurs when the brain is unable to produce insulin (de la Monte & Wands, 2005). Drugs (ie., rosiglitazone) that are used to treat type 2 diabetes are being tested to see if they help decrease or prevent Alzheimer's symptoms (De Felice, et al., 2009)

Periodontal disease as a marker for Alzheimer's

One hundred pairs of identical twins, one who had developed Alzheimer's and one who did not, were examined for differences in lifestyle. The twin who had severe periodontal disease before age 35 had a fivefold increase of developing Alzheimer's. It is thought that the periodontal disease provokes a chronic inflammatory response which may contribute to the development of Alzheimer's disease (Gatz, et al., 2006).

SYMPTOMS OF ALZHEIMER'S DISEASE

Symptoms are similar to other dementias and include:

- impaired ability to reason
- problems with memory (especially recent memory)
- eventual loss of control of the physical body and loss of the ability to speak and care for oneself

Any client who mentions memory problems severe enough to interfere with activities of daily living should have an evaluation for dementia. This evaluation can be done with a Mini-Mental Status Exam (MMSE) or a test called the 7-Minute Screen (advertised as being able to diagnose the presence of Alzheimer's with a 90% accuracy rate).

Memory difficulties often cause compliance problems with medication. This can lead to other medical problems and drug toxicities that may escalate into greater memory difficulties and even more severe medical problems.

Diagnosis of Alzheimer's disease

Usually the diagnosis of Alzheimer's disease requires the finding of characteristic "plaques and tangles" using microscopic examination of brain tissue at autopsy. It is believed that the plaques and tangles interfere with the normal functioning of nerve cells and with the production of acetylcholine. Autopsies of brains of people who had no signs of dementia have been found to have plaques and tangles.

The cause of the plaques and tangles is not fully understood, and there is no cure for Alzheimer's. Current treatments are only minimally effective in slowing the progress of the disease and there are no treatments known to reverse the symptoms.

It is only through information gained by the use of Positron Emission Tomography (PET) scans and other brain-imaging techniques, specifically functional Magnetic Resonance Imaging (fMRI), and by using quantitative EEGs (QEEGs) (Prichep, 2007), that early diagnosis has become possible. Recent studies using these techniques indicate progressive changes in the brain, particularly in the area of the hippocampus. The changes can be seen by comparing an individual's brain scans and QEEGs over time. There is hope that these techniques will lead to both earlier diagnosis and earlier treatment, and therefore to a better prognosis, for those who are at increased risk or those who show early signs of Alzheimer's disease (Fox, 2000; Fox, et al., 2001).

Treatment of Alzheimer's

Drugs currently approved by the FDA to treat dementia fall into three categories:

1. Drugs that reverse the decrease in ACh in the hippocampus (cholinergic agents such as galantamine/Reminyl and cholinesterase inhibitors such as rivastigmine/Exelon, donepezil/Aricept, tacrine/Cognex, huperzine). The most common adverse effects of these drugs are nausea, fatigue, and dizziness.

2. Drugs that increase oxygen to the brain by increasing blood flow (such as ergoloid mesylates/Hydergine).

3. Drugs that target the glutaminergic system, the N-methyl-D-aspartate (NMDA) inhibitors (such as memantine/Namenda).

ERGOLOID MESYLATES

Hydergine is the brand name for a group of compounds (ergoloid mesylates) which are believed to improve cognition by enhancing the metabolic activity of brain cells. Hydergine is widely used in countries outside the U.S. for the treatment of dementia and the cognitive deficits that may accompany aging. Hydergine is approved by the FDA for treatment of Alzheimer's disease and has been administered in the U.S. for this purpose since the 1980s. A recent review of the literature concludes that Hydergine shows significant effectiveness when compared with a placebo (although there is some skepticism among authorities in the field about the validity of this research) (Thompson, et al., 1990).

DRUGS THAT TARGET THE GLUTAMINERGIC SYSTEM

NMDA inhibitors

One theory attributes Alzheimer's disease to an over-stimulation of certain CNS nerve cells which leads to cell death. This idea has resulted in the development of drugs that work as antagonists at NMDA receptors. One FDA approved medication in this category, memantine hydrochloride/Namenda, is already on the market. Memantine seems to protect the brain from damage while still allowing normal signal transmission between cells (Winblad & Poritis, 1999). The most common adverse effects with memantine are dizziness, confusion, agitation and headache.

All of these drugs are somewhat helpful in slowing the process of dementia, but cannot stop the progress of the disease. Eventually, the decline in functioning reaches a point where the benefit from the drugs is no longer detectable.

Possible preventative measures

There is evidence that the usual measures which lead to good health (e.g., moderate exercise, good nutrition) and mental activity (such as learning something new) also support healthy aging and may possibly be helpful in slowing or preventing dementia (Cuttler & Mattson, 2006).

Studies show that sleep cycles are disrupted in people with Alzheimer's (Singer & Bahr, 2005). It is believed that regulating sleep may help to prevent dementia. Melatonin and light therapy both have been found to be helpful in this way. Because there are very few FDA-approved drugs for dementia, most of this chapter will discuss possible preventative measures and the drugs and herbal remedies that are being tested for safety and efficacy at the present time.

There is evidence to indicate that inflammatory processes are involved in the development of Alzheimer's disease. These findings make neuroinflammation a tempting target for new preventative therapies. Many current Alzheimer's disease prevention interventions employ substances that are antioxidative and anti-inflammatory. Anti-atherosclerotic diets, such as the Mediterranean diet that includes fish (n-3 polyunsaturated fatty acids), fresh fruits and vegetables, whole grains, and wine in moderation, are now recommended for the maintenence of cognitive abilities (Stanridge, 2005).

Fruit and vegetable juice

People who drank fruit or vegetable juice at least three times a week were four times less likely to develop Alzheimer's than those who did not. The study had 1800 elderly Japanese as subjects. The specific reason for this effect was not stated (Borenstein, et al., 2005).

Resveratrol/trans-3,4,5-trihydroxystilben, found in red wine

It has been documented that resveratrol, a naturally occurring substance mainly found in grapes and red wine, markedly lowers levels of amyloid-beta (a component of the plaques). Resveratrol does not inhibit amyloid production but instead promotes intracellular degradation of amyloid. This means that resveratrol may have some potential for treating Alzheimer's disease (Marambaud, et al., 2005).

Coffee

Moderate (3-5 cups/day) coffee drinkers when assessed at midlife had a lower risk of dementia (65% decrease) and less Alzheimer's disease later in life, compared with those drinking little or no coffee. This large, long-term study was adjusted for demographic, lifestyle, and vascular factors, apolipoprotein E 4 allele (a genetic factor), and depressive symptoms (Eskelinen, et al., 2009). See Chapter 6 for extensive information on caffeine.

Folate

Older people taking the recommended daily allowance (RDA) of 400 mg of folate, in food or as a supplement, appeared to have a 55% reduced risk of developing Alzheimer's when compared with those who were not getting the RDA (Corrada, 2005).

Yellow pigment in curry (curcumin)

The rate of Alzheimer's among adults 70–79 years old in India is 4.4 times less than the rate in the U.S. This has led to the idea that curcumin (a common ingredient in Southeast Asian diets) and has antioxidant and anti-inflammatory properties, may have protective and/or therapeutic effects for the elderly and those with Alzheimer's (Lim, et al., 2001).

Other possibly helpful drugs

Other drugs which may delay the onset of Alzheimer's or that have shown therapeutic value with patients already affected are:

- antioxidants (vitamin C and E, selegiline/Eldepryl, an MAOI)
- hormone replacement therapy (estrogens and/or androgens) (Yaffe, et al., 2005)
- anti-inflammatory drugs (NSAIDs, e.g. ibuprofen/Motrin) (Vlad, et al., 2008)
- neurotropic agents (human nerve growth factor)
- statin drugs (lower cholesterol) (Green, et al., 2006)
- nicotine (stimulates ACh)
- DHA (fish oil)
- phosphotidylserine/PtdSer (a fat-soluble nutrient found naturally in our bodies) (Pepeu et al., 1996)
- antiamyloid treatments (gene therapy or vaccines) (Bullock, 2002; Delagarza, 1998; Flint & van Reekum, 1998; Grundman & Thai, 2000; Pepeu, et al., 1996)
- cannabinoids (Koppel & Davies, 2008; Ramirez, et al., 2005)

DRUGS AND OTHER THERAPIES CURRENTLY BEING TESTED

A very large number of drugs are currently being tested for safety and efficacy for the treatment or prevention of Alzheimer's and other forms of dementia. It is hoped that some of these new compounds will prove to be effective and have a low toxicity. For a complete list of drugs in the pipeline and open clinical trials, see www.alz.org.

Latrepirdine

Latrepirdine/Dimebon is an antihistamine that recently had been found to have beneficial effects in neurodegenerative disease. Its mechanism of action is not known. In one study (Doody, et al., 2008) patients who received latrepirdine showed significant improvement on measures of cognition, psychiatric symptoms, and activities of daily living. In this study latrepirdine showed increasing benefits at 52 weeks. The only adverse effect reported was dry mouth. This drug is not currently available in the U.S. Recent results of a Phase III study for safety and efficacy did not find this drug at all effective (Pfizer, 2010). Even so, research using latrepirdine in combination with other cognition enhancing drugs is continuing.

Tumor Necrosis Factor (TNF) blockers: etanercept

One agent that has been approved by the FDA for the treatment of arthritis, etanercept/Enbrel, has shown effectiveness in a pilot study, of immediately reducing the symptoms of AD (Richard-Miceli & Dougados, 2001; Tobinick, et al., 2006).

Methylene blue (methylthioninium chloride)

Findings indicate that Rember, a formulation of methylene blue, works by enhancing mitochondrial function to expand the mitochondrial reserve of the brain. Adequate mitochondrial reserve is essential for preventing age-related disorders such as Alzheimer's disease. It is also believed that this compound targets the tangles of abnormal tau protein found in the brain cells of Alzheimer's patients. Basic studies suggest that Rember dissolves tau (Atamna, et al., 2007). No news or research on this drug has appeared since 2008.

Ginkgo biloba

Ginkgo biloba has been widely used outside the U.S. for many years to improve memory. Most early studies indicate significant cognitive improvement in people who have been taking ginkgo. There are adverse effects (see p. 205). However, in contrast to the earlier studies, a recent study in people with dementia who took ginkgo either for 12 or 24 weeks showed no significant effect on cognitive decline or any other measurable outcomes compared with a control group taking no medication (DeKosky, et al., 2008; Van Dongen, et al., 2000).

Other herbs being studied

Many herbs are being investigated for cognition-enhancing (nootropic) properties. Some that are under study, but are not approved by the FDA, are:

- *Bacopa monnieri*/Bacopa (Roodenrys, et al., 2002)
- *Huperzia serrata*/Huperzine A
      (Kozikowski & Tuckmantel, 1999)
- *Vinca minor* (periwinkle)/Vinpocetine
      (Singh & Dhawan, 1982; Xu, et al., 1999)
- brahmi rasayana (BR-2T) an ayurvedic
      preparation (Joshi & Parle, 2006).

Antibiotic therapy

Evidence exists that an excess of copper and zinc in the brain promotes the accumulation of beta-amyloid, which may lead to the development of the "plaques" seen in Alzheimer's. The antibiotic clioquinol, which has the ability to chelate metals (form specific molecular complexes), may facilitate removal of copper and zinc from the brain. This may lead to a reduction of amyloid deposits. It is hoped that a reduction in amyloid will lead to a decrease of some symptoms of dementia (Cuajungco, et al., 2000).

Gene therapy

There has been some success with repairing brain cells that are no longer producing acetylcholine. In this research, a gene is inserted into a brain cell enabling it to produce human nerve growth factor (NGF). NGF promotes the generation of new neurons to produce ACh which could reverse the changes caused by Alzheimer's. This research is now in Phase II clinical trials (Bakay, et al., 2002).

Enzyme-blocking therapy

Scientists have identified an enzyme, beta-secretase, which is thought to play a role in the buildup of abnormal amyloid plaques. Researchers are studying the blocking of gamma-secretase, another component in the formation of plaques. At this stage it is not known whether there will be any serious detrimental effects caused by blocking either beta or gamma secretase (Xia, 2003).

Plaque-blocking vaccine

A "vaccine" consisting of beta-amyloid protein has been shown to prevent naturally-occurring amyloid plaques from forming and eliminate pre-existing amyloid plaques in the brains of lab rats (Schenk, et al., 2001). So far, eliminating plaques has not led to a decrease in the symptoms of dementia. It is believed this is due to the disease having progressed too far, to a point where the damage is irreversible. It is hoped that with earlier intervention these drugs will be more successful. For this reason, researchers are focusing on methods of early detection and hoping to intervene in the disease process before there is too much damage.

Ampakines

The ampakines are a class of drugs which interact with glutamate receptors. Ampakines have been found to improve memory and cognition in the elderly and to increase ability to do tasks of daily living.

Giving ampakines to patients who were suffering from both schizophrenia and Alzheimer's disease has uncovered a synergistic interaction between ampakines and antipsychotic drugs. A number of ampakines are currently in clinical trials (Johnson, et al., 1999). Delays due to concerns about toxicity and drug company business policies have slowed this research.

For an extensive review of directions in research in the treatment of Alzheimer's see Klafki, et al., (2006).

Medications for agitation and depression with dementia

In the past, antipsychotic medications (see Chapter 7) were frequently used to calm patients with dementia. It has been discovered that these medications increase the risk for death in elderly patients with dementia and should not be used in this population without careful evaluation. There is now a "black box" warning on the use of antipsychotic medications for this population. It has been found that the SSRIs (see Chapter 4) are safe and effective for the agitation and depression seen in patients with dementia. Of course if the person is not responding to the SSRI it is best to discontinue the medication (Culang, et al., 2009).

Direct Relevance to Psychotherapy

Although we cannot yet do much about the consequences of dementia and its effect on memory and learning, psychotherapists can be helpful and supportive with the emotional consequences of dementia, not only with the patient, but also with the family and the care-givers. We will be called upon as sources of information and support as families make decisions as to how the person with dementia is regarded and cared for as the disease progresses. Many difficult decisions arise as the patient has less and less ability to handle the tasks of daily living, such as bathing, dressing, eating, and as the general care for the person with dementia becomes a full-time job for the care-giver. Families have to deal with many end-of-life issues, the need for conservatorship, power-of-attorney, "living wills," hospice care, legal and fiduciary issues, as well as the many family conflicts that often arise in stressful and sad situations.

Feelings of anger, frustration, and grief are inevitable and need to be processed during the course of the disease. Although most of the therapeutic work is with families and care-givers, the therapist also has to be sensitive to the mental status of the person with dementia and his or her need for emotional and medical support, particularly in the early stages of dementia when depression is common. As therapists, it is our responsibility to be realistic and well-informed about dementia, the possible options for treatment, and the resources available so that we can best assist geriatric clients and their families.

The Alzheimer's Association and the Center for Research on Aging are valuable resources for professionals, for families of patients looking for answers to questions, and for training on issues related to dementia. All clients and their families who are coping with these disorders need to be made aware of these valuable resources.

References for Chapter 10

Alzheimer's Association (2010). 800-272-3900. Retrieved from, http://www.alz.org/

Atamna, H., Nguyen, A., Schultz, C., Boyle, K., Newberry, J., Kato, H. & Ames, B. (2007). Methylene blue delays cellular senescence and enhances key mitochondrial biochemical pathways. *FASEB Journal*, 22 (3), 703.

Bakay, R., Pay, M. & Merrill, D. (2002). Growth factor gene therapy for Alzheimer's disease. *Neurosurg. Focus*, 13(5), Article 5.

Borenstein, A., Dai, Q., Wu, Y., Jackson, J. & Larson, E. (2005). Consumption of fruit and vegetable juices predicts a reduced risk of Alzheimer's disease: The Kame Project. *Alzheimer's and Dementia: J. Alzheimer's Assn.*, 1, 1, (Suppl.), S60-61.

Bullock, R. (2002). New drugs for Alzheimer's disease and other dementias. *Brit. J. Psychiatry*, 180, 135–139

Corrada, M., Kawas, C., Halldrisch, J., Muller D. & Brookmeyer, R. (2005). Reduced risk of Alzheimer's disease with high folate intake: The Baltimore Longitudinal Study of Aging. *Alzheimer's & Dementia*, 1, 11-18.

Cuajungco, K., Huang, X., Tanzi, R. & Bush, A. (2000). The Molecular Basis of Dementia, Metal chelation as a potential therapy for Alzheimer's disease. *Annals of the New York Academy of Sciences*, 920, 292–304.

Culang, M., Sneed, J., Keilp, J., Rutherford, B., Pelton, G., Devanand, D. & Roose, S. (2009). Change in cognitive functioning following acute antidepressant treatment in late-life depression. *Am. J. Geriatric Psychiatry*, 17(10), 881-88.

Cuttler, R. & Mattson, M. (2006). The adversities of aging. *Aging Res. Rev.*, 5, 221-238.

De Felice, F., Vieira, M., Bomfim, T., Decker, H., Velasco, P., Lambert, M., Viola, K., Zhao, W., Ferreira, S. & Klein, W. (2009) Protection of synapses against Alzheimer's-linked toxins: Insulin signaling prevents the pathogenic binding of A-beta oligomers. *Proc. Natl. Acad. Sci. U S A*, 106(6), 1971-6. Erratum in: *Proc. Natl. Acad. Sci. U S A*, 2009 May 5;106(18), 7678. Comment in: *Sci Signal.* 2009; 2(74), 36.

DeKosky, S., Williamson, J., Fitzpatrick, A., Kronmal, R., Ives, D., Saxton, J., Lopez, O., Burke, G., Carlson, M., Fried, L., Kuller, L., Robbins, J., Tracy, R., Woolard, N., Dunn, L., Snitz, B., Nahin, R. & Furberg, C. (2008). Ginkgo biloba for prevention of dementia: A randomized controlled trial. *JAMA,* 300(19), 2253-262.

Delagarza, V. (1998). New drugs for Alzheimer's disease. *Am. Fam. Physician,* 58(5), 1175–1182.

de la Monte, S. & Wands, J. (2005). Review of insulin and insulin-like growth factor expression, signaling, and malfunction in the central nervous system: Relevance to Alzheimer's disease. *J. Alzheimer's Dis.,* 7, 45-61.

Doody, R., Gavrilova, S., Sano, M., Thomas, R., Aisen, P., Bachurin, S., Seely, L. & Hung, D. (2008). Effect of dimebon on cognition, activities of daily living, behavior, and global function in patients with mild-to-moderate Alzheimer's disease: A randomized, double-blind, placebo-controlled study. *Lancet,* 372, 207.

Eskelinen, M., Ngandu, T., Tuomilehto, J., Soininen, H. & Kivipelto, M. (2009). Midlife coffee and tea drinking and the risk of late-life dementia: A population-based CAIDE study. *J. Alzheimer's Disease,* 16(1), 85-91.

Flint, A. & van Reekum, R. (1998). The pharmacologic treatment of Alzheimer's disease: A guide for the general psychiatrist. *Can. J. Psychiatry,* 43(7) 689–697.

Fox, N. (2000). Increased rates of atrophy in early and preclinical AD: Studies with registration of serial MRI. *Neurobiol. Aging,* 21(Suppl. 1) S74, Abstract 330.

Fox, N., Crum, W., Scahill, R. & Rossor, M. (2001). Patterns of tissue loss in degenerative dementia detected with voxel compression mapping of serial MRI. Where does atrophy in Alzheimer's disease start and how does it progress? Program and abstracts of the 17th World Congress of Neurology; June 17–22. London, UK. *Neurol. Sci.,* 187, (Suppl. 1), S116. Abstract 57.05.

Gatz, M., Mortimer, J. & Fratiglioni, L. (2006). Potentially modifiable risk factors for dementia in identical twins. *Alzheimer. Dement.,* 2, 110–117.

Green, R., McNagny, S., Jayakumar, P., Cupples, L., Benke, K. & Farrer, L. (2006). Statin use and the risk of Alzheimer's disease: The MIRAGE Study Alzheimer's & Dementia. *J. Alzheimer's Assn.,* 2(2), 96-103.

Grundman, M. & Thai, L. (2000). Treatment of Alzheimer's disease: Rationale and strategies. *Neurol. Clin.,* 18(4), 807–828.

Harold, D., Abraham, R., Hollingworth, P., Sims, R., Gerrish, A., Hamshere, M., Pahwa, J., Moskvina, V., Dowzell, K. & Williams, A. (2009). Genome-wide association study identifies variants at CLU and PICALM associated with Alzheimer's disease. *Nature Genetic.,* 10.1038/ng.440.

Johnson, S., Luu, N., Herbst, T., Knapp, R., Lutz, D., Arai, A., Rogers, G. & Lynch, G. (1999). Psychological effects of a drug that facilitates brain AMPA receptors. *J. Pharmacol. Exp. Ther.,* 289(1), 392–397.

Joshi, H. & Parle, M. (2006). Brahmi rasayana improves learning and memory in mice. *Evid. Based Complement. Alternat. Med.,* 3(1), 79–85.

Klafki, H., Staufenbiel, M., Kornhuber, J. & Wiltfang, J. (2006). Therapeutic approaches to Alzheimer's disease. *Brain,* 129(11), 2840-855.

Koppel, J. & Davies, P. (2008) Targeting the endocannabinoid system in Alzheimer's disease. *J. Alzheimers Dis.,* 15(3), 495-504.

Kozikowski, A. & Tuckmantel, W. (1999). Chemistry, pharmacology, and clinical efficacy of the Chinese nootropic agent huperzine A. *Acc. Chem. Res.,* 32, 641-650.

Lambert, J-C., Heath, S., Even, G., Campion, D., Sleegers, K., Hiltunen, M., Combarros, O., Zelenika, D., Bullido, M. & Tavernier, B. (2009). Genome-wide association study identifies variants at CLU and CR1 associated with Alzheimer's disease. *Nature Genetics,* (6 September),439, Letter.

Lim, G., Chu, T., Yang, F., Beech, W., Frautschy, S. & Cole, G. (2001).The curry spice curcumin reduces oxidative damage and amyloid pathology in an Alzheimer transgenic mouse. *J. Neuroscience,* 21(21), 8370-377.

Marambaud, P., Zhao, H. & Davies, P. (2005). Resveratrol promotes clearance of Alzheimer's disease amyloid-peptides. *J. Biol. Chem.,* 280, 37377-382.

Pepeu, G., Marconcini-Pepeu, I. & Amaducc, L. (1996). A review of phospho-tidylserine pharmacological and clinical effects: Is phosphotidylserine a drug for the aging brain? *Pharmacological Research,* 33,(2), 73–80.

Pfizer. (2010). Pfizer And Medivation Announce Results From Two Phase 3 Studies In Dimebon (latrepirdine*) Alzheimer's Disease Clinical Development Program. Retrieved March 4, 2010. http://mediaroom.pfizer.com/news/pfizer/20100303005865/en/Pfizer-Medivation-Announce-Results-Phase-3-Studies

Prichep, L. (2007). Imaging and the aging brain, Quantitative EEG and electromagnetic brain imaging in aging and in the evolution of dementia. *Annals of the New York Academy of Sciences,* 1097, 156-167.

Ramirez, B., Blázquez, C., Gómez del Pulgar, T., Guzmán, M. & de Ceballos, M. (2005). Prevention of Alzheimer's disease pathology by cannabinoids: Neuroprotection mediated by blockade of microglial activation. *J. Neurosci.,* 25(8), 1904-913.

Richard-Miceli, C. & Dougados, M. (2001). Tumour necrosis factor-alpha blockers in rheumatoid arthritis: Review of the clinical experience. *Bio. Drugs,* 15, 251-59.

Roodenrys, S., Booth, D., Buzomi, S., Phipps, A., Micallef, C. & Smoker, J. (2002). Chronic effects of Brahmi (Bacopa monnieri) on human memory. *Neuropsychopharm.,* 27, 279-81.

Schenk, D., Seubert, P. & Ciccarelli, R. (2001). Immunotherapy with beta-amyloid for Alzheimer's disease: A new frontier. *DNA Cell Biol.,* 20(11), 679–681.

Singer, C. & Bahr, A. (2005). Assessing and treating sleep disorders in patients with Alzheimer's disease. *Psychiatric Times, Special Report,* 37-40.

Singh, H. & Dhawan, B. (1982). Effect of Bacopa moniera Linn. (brahmi) extract on avoidance response in rat. *J. Ethnopharmacol.,* 5(2), 205–214.

Standridge, J. (2005). The pharmacologic prevention of Alzheimer's disease. *Alzheimer's and Dementia: J. Alzheimer's Assn.,* 1, 1, (Suppl.), S64.

Thompson, T., Filley, C., Mitchell, W., Culig, K., Lo Verde, M. & Byyny, R. (1990). Lack of efficacy of Hydergine in patients with Alzheimer's disease. *New England J. Med.,* 323, 445–448.

Tobinick, E., Gross, H., Weinberger, A. & Cohen, H. (2006). TNF-alpha modulation for treatment of Alzheimer's disease: A 6-month pilot study. *Med.Gen.Med.,* 8(2), 25.

Van Dongen, M., Van Rossum, E., Kessels, A., Seilhorst, H. & Knipschild, P. (2000). Efficacy of ginkgo for elderly people with dementia and age-associated mem-ory impairment: New results of a randomized clinical trial. *J. Am. Geriatric*

Soc., 48, 1183–1194.

Vlad, S., Miller, D., Kowall, N. & Felson, D. (2008). Protective effects of NSAIDs on the development of Alzheimer's disease. *Neurology,* 70, 1672-677.

Winblad, B. & Poritis, N. (1999). Memantine in severe dementia: The results of the M-BEST study (Benefit and Efficacy in Severely Demented Patients During Treatment with Memantine). *Int. J.Geriatric Psychiatry,* 14, 135–136.

Xia, W. (2003). Amyloid inhibitors and Alzheimer's disease. *Current Opinion Investig. Drugs,* 4(1), 55–59.

Xu, S., Gao, Z. & Weng, Z. (1999). Huperzine-A in capsules and tablets for treating patients with Alzheimer's disease. *Acta. Pharmacol. Sinica,* 20(6), 486–490.

Yaffe, K., Krueger, K., Cummings, S., Blackwell, T., Henderson, V., Sarkar, S., Ensrund, K. & Grady, D. (2005). Effect of raloxifene on prevention of dementia and cognitive impairment in older women: The multiple outcomes of raloxifene evaluation (MORE) randomized trial. *Am. J. Psychiatry,* 162, 683-90.

Chapter 11

Supplements, Herbs, & Oils

But flowers distill'd though they with winter meet,
Lose but their show; their substance still lives sweet.
William Shakespeare

The use of "supplements" for medicinal purposes increased by over 400% between 1990 and 2000 (Fugh-Berman, 2000). As of 2007, approximately 20% of people in the U.S. were using natural products for therapy (Barnes, et al., 2007). No FDA approval is required for these substances, which means that supplements do not have to be tested for safety and efficacy. Since these products are not regulated, we cannot even be certain that the label accurately reflects the contents of the

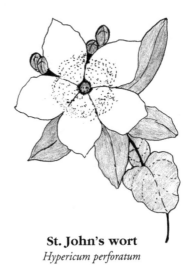

St. John's wort
Hypericum perforatum

package. ConsumerLab.com (a private company that evaluates these products) reported that 40% of the herbal preparations they tested did not meet their standards for approval primarily because they contained less of the active ingredients than the labels claimed (Burros, 2002).

The *U.S. Pharmacopoeia* (*USP*) has created a dietary supplement verification program (http://www.usp.org/) to insure that a product contains the ingredients stated in the declared amounts, that it has been screened for harmful contaminants (e.g., pesticides and heavy metals), that it has been manufactured using safe, sanitary and well-controlled procedures, and that the product will dissolve effectively to release nutrients into the body. Any manufacturer may voluntarily send in items to be screened, but it is not mandatory to do so. This information is available free on-line from www.usp.org (2010).

In addition to vitamins, minerals, and other types of supplements, more than 500 "herbal products" are currently marketed in the U.S. It is estimated that approximately 60 million Americans are using these products, primarily to treat chronic physical problems, such as joint pain and high blood pressure, as well as for psychiatric disorders, in particular sleep disorders, anxiety, and depression. This chapter only focuses on the preparations that are being used as sleep aids or to treat psychological symptoms. For extensive information see: http://www.nlm.nih.gov/medlineplus/druginfo/natural/patient.html.

If taken one at a time and not combined with each other or with other medications, these products are generally considered safe. Some have been in use in other cultures for hundreds or even thousands of years. Even so, data on these products' efficacy, adverse effects, safety, and interactions with other drugs have only recently begun to be collected in the United States.

According to Tufts Center for the Study of Drug Development, it now takes between 10 and 15 years to develop and gain FDA-approval to market a new prescription drug in the U.S. The average cost to do so is about $1.3 billion, much of which is due to the expense of clinical trials. Only three of every ten drugs that make it to the market recoup R&D costs (2010).

Because most of the alternative products are obtained naturally and cannot be patented, few companies that produce supplements are willing or able to incur this enormous expense. It is difficult for a manufacturer to commit to the huge cost of research and development if there is not enough potential profit to be gained through the use of patents to assure ownership and sole marketing rights for a substantial number of years.

Even medications approved by the FDA are sometimes found to have surprising adverse effects after they are put on the market and then taken by many thousands of people. Two well-known examples are thalidomide, which was found to cause birth defects, and various antibiotics that were later found to cause serious, and sometimes fatal, blood disorders. These same risks exist when alternative treatments are first put on the market and then taken by thousands of people.

Before taking any medication, even FDA-approved drugs, clients need to talk with their physicians and obtain as much information as possible. The longer a product has been on the market, the more that becomes known about its adverse effects and its interactions with other compounds. The physician needs to ascertain (to the extent possible) that each product does not interfere with any other drug being taken, or worsen any existing medical problem. If any type of medical procedure or surgery is planned, it is particularly important for the physician to be informed of any herbal or other type of alternative medication currently being taken (including vitamins and minerals), as these may interfere with blood clotting or interact with other drugs used during or after surgery.

Vitamins, Minerals & Other Supplements

Only one person in ten eats the recommended number of servings of fruits and vegetables each day (nine), and therefore most adults do not get the RDA of important nutrients. Many physicians advise taking a daily multivitamin/mineral supplement to make up for the nutrients that may be missing from today's typical American diet (Turnland, 1994). Malabsorption syndromes such as gluten intolerance can also lead to vitamin deficiencies.

Several minerals are known to be important for maintaining a healthy nervous system: calcium (Ca), copper (Cu), iron (Fe), phosphorus (P), potassium (K), and sodium (Na). Some (Ca, K, Na) are directly involved in the transmission of the nerve impulse.

Since we need only minute amounts of each mineral, it is best to get them through one's diet. Taking mineral supplements in pill form is usually not recommended. The main exception to this is in cases where iron-deficiency anemia has been diagnosed by a physician and iron supplements are deemed necessary (Turnland, 1994).

B COMPLEX VITAMINS

B vitamins are necessary for maintaining a healthy nervous system. They have a calming effect on some people and increase tolerance to stress. They should not be taken individually (unless recommended by a physician) as this may disturb the balance of the B vitamins to each other, causing a deficiency of one or more of the other B vitamins. Consuming alcohol may deplete the body of vitamins and can lead to a B vitamin deficiency (see chapter 3).

Vitamin B9/folate

Researchers (Taylor, et al., 2004) have shown that folate improves mood when used alone, improves response to conventional antidepressants, and may enhance the antidepressant effects of S-adenosylmethionine (SAM-e) (see page 204).

Vitamin B12/cobalamin

Vegetarians (especially vegans) may develop a B_{12} deficiency since this vitamin is primarily present in animal products (e.g., meat, milk, cheese, eggs). A deficiency in vitamin B_{12} can cause symptoms of depressed mood, weakness, and tiredness due to the disorder known as B_{12} deficiency anemia (Turnland, 1994).

Vitamin E

There is some evidence that large amounts of vitamin E can slow the progression of Alzheimer's disease. This is probably due to vitamin E's antioxidant properties (Bullock, 2002). When taken in high doses, vitamin E acts as an anticoagulant (it lengthens the time it takes for one's blood to clot). For this reason, physicians recommend discontinuing vitamin E a minimum of three weeks before any surgery.

Tryptophan and 5-hydroxytryptophan (5-HTP)

Both tryptophan and 5-HTP are amino acid precursors to the neurotransmitter serotonin (see Appendix C). Serotonin has a role in depression and anxiety. More research has been done with 5-HTP than with tryptophan. Researchers have found that 5-HTP is an effective agent for the treatment of anxiety and panic symptoms (Soderpalm & Engel, 1990). In people with chronic anxiety 5-HTP may be taken daily without causing excessive sedation and can be taken at bedtime to improve the quality of sleep in patients who complain of insomnia (Lake, 2008).

DEHYDROEPIANDROSTERONE (DHEA)

DHEA has been shown to be neuroprotective, to stimulate neural growth, and to have antagonistic effects on oxidants and glucocorticoids (Maninger, et al., 2009). In one study, the neurosteroid DHEA was added to the regular medication regimen of patients with chronic schizophrenia and prominent negative symptoms. Patients receiving the DHEA supplement had a significant improvement in mood (Rabkin, et al., 2000). In one small study with depressed patients, DHEA enhanced sexual functioning and decreased the severity of the depression (Schmidt, et al., 2005).

OMEGA-3 FATTY ACIDS

In addition to the many reported benefits to the cardiovascular system from the use of omega-3 fatty acids, there is strong evidence to support its use for the treatment of depression (Kraguljac, et al., 2009). Omega-3s are abundant in seafood, especially in oily fish like tuna, salmon, and sardines. In countries such as Japan, where fish is a mainstay of the average diet, rates of both major depression and post-partum depression are very low (Hibbeln, 1998). There is also evidence that if omega-3 fatty acids are taken in higher doses than the amounts used for unipolar depression, there is improvement in both the manic and the depressive symptoms of bipolar disorder (Calabrese, et al., 1999; Frangou, et al., 2006; Stoll, 1999). The only adverse effect noted was mild GI upset in about 25% of those treated. The specific mechanism of action is unknown but is believed to be connected to the action of the monoamine neurotransmitters.

S-ADENOSYLMETHIONINE (SAM-e)

SAM-e was isolated in 1952 and has been found to be present in all living cells. It is referred to as a "nutraceutical," a natural product that promotes good health and well-being. SAM-e is formed from the combination of adenosine triphosphate/ATP and the amino acid methionine. It is thought to enhance DA and 5-HT metabolism, and to repair the myelin which surrounds some nerve cells.

SAM-e is being used to treat depression. A meta-analysis of over 1,000 patients found that SAM-e was 17% to 38% better than placebo, and elicited a faster response than the antidepressant drug imipramine/Tofranil (Chiaie & Pancheri, 2002).

Cautions on the use of SAM-e

SAM-e can potentiate other antidepressants and therefore should not be taken along with other antidepressant medications. As with other antidepressants, it can induce a manic episode in people with bipolar disorder. It may decrease fertility in women. The active ingredients in SAM-e tend to break down rapidly, so the dose indicated on the label may not accurately reflect the contents of the tablets (Bottiglieri, 1997).

Herbal Remedies for Psychological Purposes

Herbal products have been widely used outside the U.S. for centuries, and in the past few years their use has fueled a major growth industry here. Surveys indicate that one in three Americans have used herbal remedies.

Most of these products consist of a specific part of a plant, or are made from an extract derived from part of a plant. Because some plants are composed of hundreds of different and many potentially active ingredients, it is frequently difficult to determine what the specific active compound or compounds are, and also to determine the exact amount needed for effectiveness. These factors make controlled studies of herbal remedies, where the dose of active ingredient needs to be kept constant and compared with placebo, difficult and rare.

GINKGO

Ginkgo is primarily used as a cognition-enhancing drug. It has been evaluated for this use in Alzheimer's disease, and most studies have shown that there is cognitive improvement if ginkgo is taken for three to twelve months (see Chapter 10). Some people show improvement after only one month of treatment. The improvement has been evaluated using objective tests for cognition. It is thought that ginkgo exerts its effect primarily by its ability to dilate blood vessels, and that cognition is improved

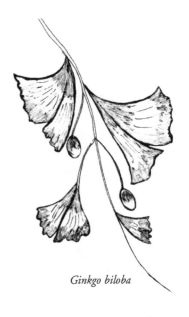

Ginkgo biloba

because the blood supply throughout the brain increases. Effectiveness is equivocal since one large placebo controlled study showed no meaningful measurable effect on cognition (Van Dongen, et al., 2000).

Adverse effects of ginkgo

There are few adverse effects associated with the use of ginkgo. Those most frequently seen are headache, sensitivity to light, and gastrointestinal problems.

Ginkgo inhibits platelet aggregation, resulting in an increase in clotting time and an increased risk of excessive bleeding. For this reason, it is not recommended for concurrent use with anticoagulants. Due to the increased risk of hemorrhage, people with diabetes and hypertension should avoid ginkgo. There is evidence that its use may increase the frequency of headaches in people who suffer from migraines (Vale, 1998).

GINSENG

Ginseng (*Panax ginseng*) and Siberian ginseng (*Eleutherococcus senticosus*) are believed to improve mood, enhance energy, and reduce stress (Pavlovich, 1999). Studies have been done comparing ginseng to placebo, with contradictory findings. This may be due to the variability of the active ingredient in different ginseng preparations. In addition, at least 20 different ginsenosides (ginseng alkaloids) have been identified; each may have different pharmacological activity, and some of the activities may counteract each other.

Some effects of ginseng

- corticosteroid-like activity
- a decrease in blood glucose
- inhibition of platelet aggregation
- estrogenic effect (generates estrogen)
- can produce vaginal bleeding and swollen breasts

One case report indicated a negative result due to the interaction of ginseng and phenelzine, an MAO inhibitor. A depressed patient experienced mania, insomnia, and headache after taking ginseng and phenelzine (Jones & Runikis, 1987).

KAVA

Kava *(Piper methysticum)* is used mainly for reduction of anxiety and as a sleep-inducing agent. A meta-analysis found kava to be effective in reducing anxiety (Pittler & Ernst, 2000). Positive effects were seen as early as one week after treatment. Kava was superior to placebo in all of the reviewed trials. It is believed that kava works by blocking norepinephrine reuptake, suppressing the release of glutamate, and increasing GABA receptor density (Pittler & Ernst, 2000).

Adverse effects of kava

There were a few complaints of restlessness, mild GI upset and tremor. It is believed that ingredients in kava act as skeletal muscle relaxants and as anticonvulsants and may potentiate other sedative drugs. A comatose state was reported in a patient who took kava and was already taking alprazolam/Xanax (a BzRA). The coma occurred three days after taking kava. The use of multiple drugs made the interpretation of the interactions inconclusive. The patient recovered without significant problems (Almeida & Grimsley, 1996; Pittler & Ernst, 2000). Twenty-five cases of liver toxicity that occurred in Switzerland and Germany have been reported to the FDA. It is believed that this was due to a problem with one batch of kava.

In 2002 the FDA issued a consumer advisory stating that kava products may be associated with severe liver injury and that patients with liver problems should consult a physician before taking kava-containing products (Consumer Advisory on kava, 2002). It is unclear whether the toxicity was due to the kava or to other factors.

ST. JOHN'S WORT (SJW)

St. John's wort *(Hypericum perforatum)* is believed to block reuptake of norepinephrine and serotonin. It has been used for many years as an antidepressant in Germany, where clinical trials have indicated efficacy comparable to TCAs (Linde, et al., 1996). SJW has recently gained popularity and is now the most widely used herbal compound for depression in the United States (Bilia, et al., 2002). There have been many recent studies comparing the efficacy of SJW to placebo, SSRIs, and TCAs; most show SJW to be as effective, with fewer adverse effects, as these drugs are in treating mild to moderate depressions (Bilia, et al., 2002; Linde, et al., 1996). However, one recent, carefully-controlled study found that the effectiveness of taking SJW for major depression was not significantly greater than taking a placebo (Shelton, et al., 2001). SSRIs are also not very effective for major depression.

Treatment of somatoform disorders with SJW

Researchers have found that SJW is effective for the treatment of somatoform disorders independent of depressed mood. They concluded that the specific advantages of SJW are a good safety profile, absence of any sedating effect, and a rapid onset of response (Voltz, et al., 2002).

Adverse effects of SJW

The most frequently seen adverse effects are mild GI symptoms and fatigue. People with epilepsy should consult their physicians before taking SJW, since there have been reports of an increase in seizure activity when taking the drug. SJW may increase the frequency and duration of migraine headaches. Photosensitivity has been reported in light-sensitive people taking high doses of SJW. This effect was reversed when SJW was discontinued. Excessive sedation was reported in one elderly subject who was also taking paroxetine. It is recommended that SJW not be used in conjunction with MAO inhibitors or with foods containing tyramine (see p. 66).

Since SJW is reported to interact with a number of other medications, it is advisable to use caution when it is taken in combination with any other compound. This is particularly relevant for drugs that may have a stimulating effect such as:

- disulfiram/Antabuse
- caffeine
- antidepressants
- immunosuppressive drugs
- theophylline (an asthma medication)
- over-the-counter cough and cold medicines
- any other herbal products (Linde, et al., 1996)

WARNING: There is evidence that St. John's wort decreases the effectiveness of birth control pills.

PYCNOGENOL

Pycnogenol/pine bark extract, was tested as a cognition-enhancer on healthy elderly individuals using a double-blind, placebo-controlled design, with 101 elderly participants (60-85 years) for a treatment period of three months. The pycnogenol group displayed statistically significant improved working memory relative to the control group (Ryan, et al., 2008).

RESVERATROL

Resveratrol, (trans-3,4,5-trihydroxystilbene) is a product extracted from red wine. Resveratrol is found both in grapes and in red wine. Large doses of it markedly lowers the levels of amyloid-B. This suggests that this natural compound may have therapeutic potential in the treatment of Alzheimer's disease (Marambaud, et al., 2005). Resveratrol has been demonstrated to be a potent antioxidant (about 20–50 times stronger than vitamin C) and to act synergistically with vitamin C, enhancing the effects of each (Marambaud, et al., 2005).

VALERIAN

This herb *(Valeriana officinalis)* works immediately to reduce feelings of nervousness. It improves the quality of sleep by decreasing both sleep latency and nocturnal awakenings due to anxiety. Its effect is believed to be due to its interaction with GABA receptors (Donath, et al., 2000).

Adverse effects of valerian

Since valerian causes drowsiness, one should not drive or operate dangerous machinery after taking it. Some people have a drug hangover in the morning after having taken it to help with sleep. As with all sedatives, valerian should not be used while taking any other sleep or antianxiety medications (Santillo, 1984).

Essential Oils (Aromatherapy)

This section is intended to be used as a quick-reference guide for the therapist who has clients who are using aromatherapy. There are many books on aromatherapy and clients need to educate themselves in the appropriate uses of, and any dangers associated with, each oil.

Aromatherapy practitioners describe their practice as "the art of healing with the concentrated extracts from plants, herbs, and flowers" that are called "essential oils." The aromas of these oils are said to relieve stress, lessen depression and mental fatigue, as well as decrease a variety of physical ailments. The popularity of aromatherapy is growing by proverbial leaps and bounds, but how (or if) it works is yet to be scientifically proven (Dunn, et al., 1995).

Essential Oils for Psychological Purposes

Bergamot – treats depression, relieves anxiety

Blue Tansy – reduces stress, increases feelings of well-being

Celery – sedates

Chamomile – calms, reduces stress, irritability & depression

Citrus – relaxes and calms

Clary Sage – helps with symptoms of PMS, relaxes muscles, calms

Clove – treats symptoms of fatigue

Geranium – sedates, treats nervousness

Lavender – reduces headaches, relieves insomnia, reduces symptoms of PMS, reduces stress

Lemon grass – calms

Marjoram – calms, warms, soothes

Melaleuca – calms jangled nerves, relieves pain

Melissa – treats depression

Mint – clears the mind

Neroli – treats depression & anxiety

Orange – lifts spirits

Patchouli – relaxes

Pennyroyal – stimulates

Peppermint – improves mental acuity, decreases fatigue

Rose – calms nerves, assuages anger

Rosemary – clears the mind, energizes, helps memory

Rosewood – clears the head

Sage – relaxes

Sandalwood – calms nerves, relieves anxiety

Tangerine – lifts spirits

Thyme – stimulates the brain

Turkish rose – stimulates, elevates the mind

Wintergreen – stimulates

Ylang ylang – relieves tension, soothes, helps with PMS

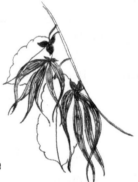

Ylang ylang
Cananga odorata

Table 11.1

WARNING: These oils are NOT TO BE TAKEN INTERNALLY. If irritation develops the use of the oil should be discontinued immediately.

Route of administration

The sense of smell is believed to be the most evocative of all the senses. The theoretical basis for the effectiveness of aromatherapy is that a connection exists between the sense of smell and the brain which can promote relaxation, increase energy, and restore balance to the mind. Aromatherapists believe that these scents work by influencing the limbic area of the brain to balance the nervous system, calm the emotions, and bolster the individual's ability to cope with stress (Green & Keville, 1995).

All of these oils can be diluted in water and used as room-misters. Putting a few drops of oil in a glass of water for misting is enough to get a pleasant scent. A few drops can be put on a handkerchief to carry and inhale throughout the day, or placed on one's pillow at bedtime (Rose, 1992).

Adverse reactions to essential oils

Some essential oils irritate the eyes and other mucous membranes; they are not to be applied directly to the skin without being diluted. A patch test for allergy is generally recommended before using any of these oils (Green & Keville, 1995; Jackson & Teague, 1975; Rose, 1992).

Direct Relevance to Psychotherapy

All of the substances discussed in this chapter can be obtained with relative ease and little expense. Most people consider these products to be safe for self-medication, and many clients do not think of them as "drugs" and therefore do not mention using them to their psychotherapist or their psychiatrist. As the popularity of these products grows, the incidence of adverse effects and interactions with other drugs will also increase. It is important that the psychotherapist ask if the client is using any herbal or "alternative" products (supplements, vitamins, or minerals) in addition to any prescription or illicit drugs.

The herbs and other products discussed here are medicinal agents and have psychoactive effects. The psychotherapist needs to caution clients about possible drug interactions. The therapist may be the first person to observe any overdose or adverse effect from these products. The FDA now maintains a database on adverse effects associated with herbal use that can be accessed at http://vm.cfsan.fda.gov/.

References for Chapter 11

Almeida, J. & Grimsley, E. (1996). Coma from the health food store: Interaction between kava and alprazolam. *Annals of Internal Medicine*, 125, 940–941.

Barnes, P., Bloom, B. & Nahin, R. (2007.) *Complementary and Alternative Medicine Use Among Adults and Children.* United States. Division of Health Interview Statistics, National Center for Health Statistics

Bilia, A., Gallori, S. & Vincieri, F. (2002). St. John's wort and depression: Efficacy, safety and tolerability-an update. *Life Sci.*, 70(26), 3077-096.

Bottiglieri, T. (1997). Ademetionine (S-adenosylmethionine) neuropharmacology: Implications for drug therapies in psychiatric and neurological disorders. *Expert Opinion in Investigational Drugs*, 6, 417–426.

Bullock, R. (2002). New drugs for Alzheimer's disease and other dementias. *Brit. J. of Psychiatry*, 180, 135–139.

Burros, M. (2002). Eating well: It's on the label but is it in the tablet? *NY Times*, January 2.

Calabrese, J., Rapport, D. & Shelton, M. (1999). Fish oils and bipolar disorder: A promising but untested treatment. *Arch. Gen. Psychiatry*, 56, 413–416.

Chiaie, R. & Pancheri, P. (2002). Efficacy and tolerability of oral and intramuscular S-adenosyl-L-methionine 1,4-butanedisulfonate (SAMe) in the treatment of major depression: Comparison with imipramine in 2 multicenter studies. *Am. J. Clin. Nutr.*, 76(Suppl.), 1172S–1176S.

Consumer Advisory on kava. (2002). http://www.cfsan.fda.gov/~dms/addskava.html.

Donath, F., Quispe, K., Maurer, A., Fietze, I. & Roots, I. (2000). Critical evaluation of the effect of valerian extract on sleep structure and sleep quality. *Pharmacopsychiatry*, 33, 47–53.

Dunn, C., Sleep, J. & Collett, D. (1995). Sensing an improvement: An experimental study to evaluate the use of aromatherapy, massage, and periods of rest in an intensive care unit. *J. Adv. Nursing*, 21, 34–40.

Frangou, S., Lewis, M. & McCrone, P. (2006). Efficacy of ethyl-eicosapentaenoic acid in bipolar depression: Randomized double-blind placebo-controlled study. *Brit. J. of Psychiatry*, 188, 46–50.

Fugh-Berman, A. (2000). Herb-drug interactions. *Lancet*, 355, 134–138.

Green, M. & Keville, K. (1995). *Aromatherapy: A Complete Guide to the Healing Art.* Santa Cruz, CA: Crossing Press.

Hibbeln, J. (1998). Fish consumption and major depression. *Lancet*, 351(9110), 1213.

Jackson, M. & Teague, T. (1975). *The Handbook of Alternatives to Chemical Medicine.* Berkeley, CA: Lawton-Teague Publications.

Jones, B. & Runikis, A. (1987). Interaction of ginseng with phenelzine. *J. Clinical Psychopharm.*, 7, 201–202.

Kraguljac, N., Montori, V., Pavuluri, M., Chai, H., Wilson, B. & Unal, S. (2009). Efficacy of omega-3 fatty acids in mood disorders-a systematic review and meta-analysis. *Psychopharmacol. Bull.*, 42(3), 39-54.

Lake, J. (2008). Integrative management of anxiety. *Psychiatric Times*, January, 13, 14-16.

Linde, K., Ramirez, G., Mulrow, C., Pauls, A., Weidenhammer, W. & Melchart, D. (1996). St. John's wort for depression: An overview and meta-analysis of randomized clinical trials. *British Med. Journal*, 313, 253–258.

Maninger, N., Wolkowitz. O., Reus, V., Epel, E. & Mellon, S. (2009). Neurobiological and neuropsychiatric effects of dehydroepiandrosterone (DHEA) and DHEA sulfate (DHEAS). *Front. Neuroendocrinol.*, 30(1), 65-91.

Marambaud, P., Zhao, H. & Davies, P. (2005). Resveratrol promotes clearance of Alzheimer's disease amyloid-B peptides. *J. Biological Chemistry*, 280, 37377-382.

Pavlovich N. (1999). Herbal remedies: The natural approach to combating stress. *J. Perianesth. Nurs.*, 14(3), 134-8.

Pittler, M. & Ernst, E. (2000). Efficacy of kava extract for treating anxiety: Systemic review and meta-analysis. *J. Clinical Psychopharm.*, 20, 84–89.

Rabkin, J., Ferrando, S., Wagner, G. & Rabkin, R. (2000). DHEA treatment for HIV+ patients: Effects on mood, androgenic and anabolic parameters. *Psychoneuroendocrin.*, 25(1), 53–68.

Rose, J. (1992). *The Aromatherapy Book: Applications and Inhalations.* Berkeley, CA: North Atlantic Books.

Ryan, J., Croft, K., Mori, T., Wesnes, K., Spong, J., Downey, L., Kure, C., Lloyd, J. & Stough C. (2008). An examination of the effects of the anti-oxidant Pycnogenol on cognitive performance, serum lipid profile, endocrinological and oxidative stress biomarkers in an elderly population. *J. Psychopharmacol.*, 22(5), 553-62.

Santillo, H. (1984). *Natural Healing with Herbs.* Prescott Valley, Arizona: HOHM Press.

Schmidt, P., Daly, R., Bloch, M., Smith, M. & Rubinow, D.(2005). Dehydroepiandrosterone monotherapy in midlife-onset major and minor depression. *Arch. Gen. Psychiatry*, 62, 154-162.

Shelton, R., Keller, M., Gelenberg, A., Dunner, D., Hirschfeld, R., Thase, M., Russell, J., Lydiard, R., Crits-Cristoph, P., Gallop, R., Todd, L., Hellerstein, D., Goodnick, P., Keitner, G., Stahl, S. & Halbreich, U. (2001). Effectiveness of St. John's Wort in major depression: A randomized clinical trial. *JAMA*, 285(15), 1978–1986.

Soderpalm, B. & Engel, J. (1990). Serotonergic involvement in conflict behavior. *Eur. Neuropsychopharm.*, 1, 7-13.

Stoll, A. (1999). Omega-3 fatty acids in bipolar disorder: A preliminary, double blind, placebo controlled trial. *Arch. Gen. Psych.*, 56(5), 407–412.

Taylor, M., Carney, S., Goodwin, G. & Geddes, J. (2004). Folate for depressive disorders: Systematic review and meta-analysis of randomized controlled trials. *J. Psychopharm.*, 18(2), 251–256.

Tufts Ctr. for Study of Drug Development. Retrieved January 30, 2010 http://csdd.tufts.edu/NewsEvents/

Turnland, J. (1994). Future directions for establishing mineral/trace element requirements. *J. Nutr.,* 124(9 Suppl.), 1765S–1770S.

U.S. Pharmacopoeia. (2010). Retrieved January 24, 2010, http://www.usp.org/

Vale, S. (1998). Subarachnoid hemorrhage associated with ginkgo biloba. *Lancet,* 352–356.

Van Dongen, M., Van Rossum, E., Kessels, A., Seilhorst, H. & Knipschild, P. (2000). Efficacy of ginkgo for elderly people with dementia and age-associated memory impairment: New results of a randomized clinical trial. *J. American Geriatric Society,* 48, 1183–1194.

Voltz, H., Murck, H., Kaspar, S. & Moller, H. (2002). St. John's Wort extract (LI 160) in somatoform disorders: Results of a placebo controlled trial. *Psychopharmacol.,* 164, 294–300.

Appendix A

The Nerve Cell & the Brain

This section is intended to provide psychotherapists, whose training typically does not include advanced courses in biochemistry and anatomy, with a simplified frame of reference to the underpinnings of modern psychopharmacology. It is the specific purview and responsibility of psychiatrists, who do have medical training and a thorough understanding of neurochemistry and the mechanisms of action for the psychoactive drugs, to determine which medication is best for each individual patient.

Structure of the Nerve Cell

Pharmacological treatment of psychological problems is based on the current understanding of the biochemical processes in the central nervous system (CNS), in particular, the use of drugs that influence neuromodulators, neurotransmitters, receptors and other substances and processes that affect nerve cells. These medications target various parts of the transmitter systems to cause changes in the CNS. These changes ultimately affect cognition, emotions, and behavior.

The nerve cell (neuron) is the basic unit of the nervous system (See Figures A1, The Neuron, and C1, The Synapse). The main components of the nerve cell are:

Axon: This is the structure along which nerve impulses are transmitted to presynaptic terminals. (See Fig. A1.)

COMT: Catechol-O-methyltransferase is an enzyme present in the synaptic cleft. (See Fig. C1.)

Dendrites: These are branching structures designed to receive impulses from adjacent nerve cells. (See Fig. C1.)

MAO: Monoamine oxidase is an enzyme present in the presynaptic terminal. (See Fig. C1.)

Myelin sheath: This covers the axon in some nerve cells. Impulses travel more quickly in myelinated nerve cells. (See Fig. A1.)

Nodes of Ranvier: These are pores in the myelin sheath that allow the impulse to "jump" along the axon from one node to the next by a process called "saltation." It is at these nodes where charged particles (ions) pass through the cell membrane, allowing the impulse to travel down the axon very rapidly. (See Fig. A1.)

Presynaptic terminal: This structure contains the synaptic vesicles. (See Fig. C1.)

Soma (or cell body): This contains the nucleus and the organelles that synthesize and package protein (e.g., Golgi apparatus, endoplasmic reticulum, mitochondria). (See Fig. A1.)

Synaptic cleft: The space between nerve cells where transmitter substances make contact with receptors. (See Fig. C1.)

Synaptic vesicles: Sites where transmitter substances are stored and protected from enzymatic degradation by monoamine oxidase (MAO). (See Fig. C1.)

The Neuron

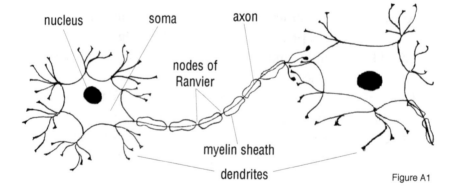

Figure A1

Glial Cells

Glial cells (see Fig. B1) are another type of cell found in the nervous system. These cells function as structural support and nutrition for neurons. They also produce myelin, and are an important component of the blood-brain barrier. Glial cells are now known to interact with transmitter substances.

The "white matter" in the brain is composed of nerve fibers coated with myelin; "gray matter" is composed of nerve fibers that are not coated with myelin. The myelin forms a fatty sheath around the nerve fiber which makes it appear white.

Transmission of the Nerve Impulse

When a nerve cell is in a "resting" state, the concentration of sodium ions (Na^{+1}) is high extracellularly (outside the cell), and low intracellularly (inside the cell). Potassium (K^{+1}) has the opposite concentration (low outside, high inside). Chlorine (Cl^{-1}) is largely extracellular, and its charge is balanced by negatively charged amino acids and proteins inside the cell. Positively charged calcium ions (Ca^{+2}) exist in free form in the cytoplasm, and these have a major role in control of many cellular functions (e.g., the activation of enzymes, and the release of compounds from synaptic vesicles). Most intracellular Ca^{+2} is sequestered in organelles within the cytoplasm, such as the endoplasmic reticulum and mitochondria, keeping the concentration of free Ca^{+2} very low. When the concentration of free Ca^{+2} rises, the processes that are dependent on free Ca^{+2} are initiated. (See Fig. A2.)

Unequal distribution of ions across cell membranes results in a "resting membrane potential" (the interior of the cell is negatively charged relative to its exterior). Neuronal firing requires a change in this resting potential. A decrease in this potential leads to depolarization. The interior of the cell becomes less negative with respect to the extracellular space; this makes the cell more likely to fire, therefore this process is considered "excitatory." An increase in potential (i.e., the interior of the cell becomes even more negatively charged) is termed "hyperpolarization." This process makes the cell less likely to fire, and is therefore termed "inhibitory."

Distribution of Ions

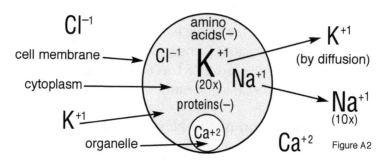

Figure A2

One way a nerve cell's membrane-potential is regulated is through ion channels. These channels depend on glycoprotein molecules (receptors) that traverse the membrane. Changes in the structure of these protein molecules cause an opening and closing of pores through which certain ions can pass. Unique properties of these glycoproteins allow for selection of ions and specific circumstances under which the channel will open. The "open" state of the channel has a specific time-course and conductance. A channel may have more than one open state (time-course and conductance can differ for the same channel).

Certain channels, called "ligand-gated channels," are closely linked to receptors and open when a specific neurotransmitter or neuro-modulator binds to the receptor. Others, designated "voltage-gated channels," respond to the degree of membrane polarization.

Specific inhibitory or excitatory neurotransmitters bind to receptor molecules. A transmitter substance, depending on the location within the brain, may be either excitatory and inhibitory. The binding leads to a change in ion conductance, or to the activation of a "second messenger" within the cell, the transmitter substance itself being the "first messenger." Activation of the second messenger system can have several effects, including the activation of enzymes that manufacture neuronal proteins, an alteration of membrane conductance, or a change in rate of protein synthesis.

Summary

Transmission of the nerve impulse is an electro-chemical phenomenon. The cell is depolarized by a flow of ions from one side of the membrane to the other, generating a charge or current that then passes down the axon. When the impulse arrives at the nerve cell terminal, it stimulates release of substances from synaptic vesicles. Transmitter substances are then released into the synaptic cleft (space between nerve cells), where transmitters contact receptors on the cell membrane of the dendrites of the next nerve cell.

There are many examples where neurons release and receive transmitters in regions that lack the specialization of the classical nerve synapse. Nevertheless, the simplified concept described here, that a transmitter released from a presynaptic cell contacts a postsynaptic receptor which then recognizes the transmitter and responds, remains useful to an understanding of most nerve-cell functions.

The interaction of a transmitter substance with a specific receptor will ultimately lead to either depolarization (firing) or to hyperpolarization (inhibition) of the next nerve cell. It is important to realize that at any one time each nerve cell is receiving input from many (probably thousands) of adjacent nerve cells. The nerve cell essentially "sums up" all of the information it is receiving, and depending upon the net result of the summation, the next neuron will either fire or be inhibited.

Please be aware that this description is a simplified version of the extremely complex processes involved in nerve cell transmission. The understanding of exactly what goes on at the synapse is beyond the scientific knowledge gained from current technology. As more is learned, the details of this process become more complex.

Appendix B
Studying the Brain

There are many obstacles to doing research on the central nervous system. The first, and most obvious, is that the brain is enclosed in the skull. This makes physical access to CNS neurons very difficult. The second major obstacle is the filtering system known as the blood-brain barrier (BBB).

The Blood-Brain Barrier

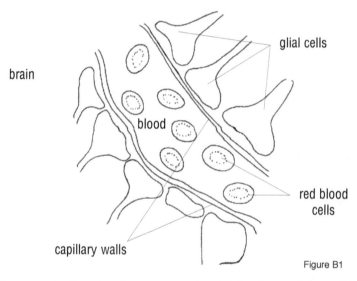

Figure B1

Studying metabolism in the organs outside the brain is possible by simply obtaining a sample of blood from a vein, usually in the arm. One can be relatively certain that the blood sample is representative of venous blood throughout the body. The blood's chemical profile can be analyzed and accurate deductions made regarding metabolic processes taking place in various organs (e.g., liver, kidney). Unfortunately, this method does not work for obtaining information about metabolism inside the brain because the BBB acts as a filter for many chemicals and compounds. This barrier is made up of capillaries that are packed tightly together and covered by a fatty sheath. This sheath is produced by the astrocyte type of glial cell. (Figure B1.)

All the blood that enters and leaves the brain must pass through this filter. The pores in the capillaries are very small, making it difficult for large molecules to enter the brain, and the fatty makeup of the sheath makes it difficult for water-soluble molecules to get through. Therefore, a blood sample taken from the arm does not reflect the chemical composition of the blood in the brain. The BBB protects the brain but at the same time makes the study of brain biochemistry and metabolism very difficult.

Scanning Techniques

Technological advances such as MRI and PET (see below) scans are facilitating exploration and understanding of brain metabolism. An American chemist and a British physicist, Paul C. Lauterbur and Peter Mansfield, were awarded the 2003 Nobel Prize for their work in the early 1970s that resulted in the development of MRI technology. This has led the way to recent advances in understanding the CNS.

Magnetic resonance imaging (MRI)

This technique is possible because the water atoms in the body can be lined up with magnets and moved with radio signals. First, all the water molecules in the body are lined up in a north-south direction. A radio signal then is used to move the water molecules away from their north-south orientation. The energy required to move the molecules varies depending upon the density of the structures in the body. This variance is analyzed and converted to digital images that represent anatomy.

Functional magnetic resonance imaging (fMRI)

This refers to the process of taking MRIs at various times (e.g., while in a psychotic state) and comparing these MRIs with those taken while in a different state (e.g., non-psychotic) to see which parts of the brain show changes.

The Limbic System

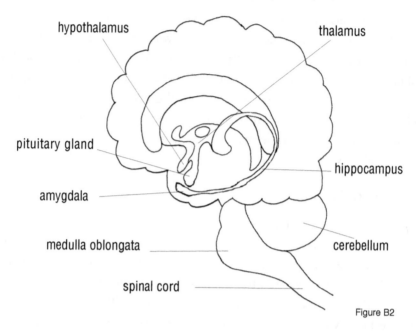

hypothalamus

thalamus

pituitary gland

hippocampus

amygdala

medulla oblongata

cerebellum

spinal cord

Figure B2

Positron emission tomography (PET)

PET scans facilitate the comparison of the degree of metabolic activity between different areas of the brain and the tracking of metabolic changes over time. This is useful for observing the progression of a disease (like Alzheimer's), the influences of various psychoactive medications on the brain, and changes in a subject's brain activity while looking at or thinking about different things. PET scans also enable comparisons of brain activity between people who have been diagnosed with a mental disorder, and those who have not.

PET and MRI scans are still being refined to yield more detailed and specific information. With these techniques it is becoming possible to label, localize, and map various neurotransmitters and neuromodulators, get more information about how they function, observe the progression of diseases such as Parkinson's and Alzheimer's, and note changes that may occur with the use of various psychoactive medications or therapeutic techniques.

Prior to the development of modern neuroimaging techniques like MRI, fMRI, and PET scans, mapping of the brain was done after autopsy by dissecting the brains of cadavers and therefore did not yield information about what was occurring in the brain of a living person. The recent advances in the understanding of the central nervous system are largely due to development of these new scanning techniques.

It is important to remember that these techniques do not provide information at the microscopic level of detail required for a specific understanding of how transmitter substances interact with receptors and how these interactions lead to our mental processes, feeling, and behaviors. Although new discoveries are constantly being made, our understanding of what goes on at the synapse is still very theoretical.

Appendix C

Transmitter Substances

Transmitter substances are molecules that relay information from the end of one nerve cell across the synaptic cleft to the receptors of the next nerve cell. Some substances that were initially called "neurotransmitters" are now being called "neuromodulators."

A neuromodulator is a chemical that modulates neuronal transmission that is primarily facilitated by some other neurotransmitter. A neuromodulator can make receptors either more or less sensitive to a neurotransmitter. Norepinephrine (NE), dopamine (DA), and serotonin (5-HT) are now considered neuromodulators to the amino acid neurotransmitters (primarily GABA and glutamate) (Gainetdihov, et al., 1999; Gladwell & Coote, 1999; Holden, 2003).

Central Nervous System Transmitter Substances

ACETYLCHOLINE (ACH)

Acetylcholine (ACh) was the first neurotransmitter to be identified. It was initially found in the peripheral nervous system (PNS), where it is the major neurotransmitter at the neuromuscular junction. ACh is also present in large amounts in the brain, with the highest concentrations found in the cerebral cortex and the caudate nucleus. ACh is also present in the basal ganglia, where it plays a role in the mediation of movement. When the balance between ACh and DA is disturbed, various movement disorders occur. Examples of this are the extrapyramidal syndrome (EPS) sometimes seen with antipsychotic medications, and the problems with movement seen with Parkinson's disease. ACh is involved in other processes such as:

- mood
- learning
- memory
- attention
- REM sleep
- behavioral arousal

ACh is involved in Alzheimer's disease, and in the negative symptoms of schizophrenia (Grundman & Thai, 2000).

Amino Acid Transmitters

Amino acids are very abundant as neurotransmitters in the brain, and can be found at about 90% of CNS transmitting sites. Neurons also use amino acids to make proteins and other neurotransmitters. Some amino acids (e.g., glutamate and aspartate) are usually excitatory, while others (e.g., GABA and glycine) are usually inhibitory.

Aspartate & glutamate

The amino acids aspartate and glutamate are the main excitatory transmitters in the CNS. Glutamate is replacing dopamine as the current focus of psychopharmacology research. Drugs that act on the glutamate system are being tested for the treatment of anxiety disorders, depression, schizophrenia, and addiction (Holden, 2003).

Gamma-aminobutyric acid (GABA)

GABA, which is thought to be the main inhibitory amino acid transmitter in the CNS, has been investigated quite extensively. Much of the research has been done on the role of GABA receptors in the action of the BzRAs. Neurons that use GABA as their transmitting agent function primarily as neurons that connect many areas of the brain. Two types of GABA receptors are GABA/A and GABA/B. In the brain, GABA/A receptors are directly coupled to chloride ion channels. After activation by GABA/A, the channel becomes permeable to chloride ions, and the neuron becomes hyperpolarized (inhibited). This inhibition seems to lead to a decrease in neuronal activity and a decrease in anxiety (Johansen, 1992).

Monoamine Transmitters (DA, NE, 5-HT)

Though less abundant in amount than the amino acid transmitters, these substances are very potent in their activity. The monoamines are thought to mainly modulate or "fine tune" the actions of the amino acid NTs, GABA, and glutamate. It is known that each monoamine transmitter has many subtypes and receptor types that affect different processes and areas of the CNS.

Dopamine (DA)

Large amounts of dopamine can be found in the nerve cells that terminate in the basal ganglia, frontal cortex, and limbic system. These nerve cells have their cell bodies in the substantia nigra of the brain stem and in the limbic system (Fig. B2). There is evidence that DA can be both excitatory and inhibitory. DA has a role in:

- emotional reactions
- schizophrenia
- normal movement
- thought processes
- addictions
- Parkinson's disease

Drugs have not yet been developed that target only one part of the brain, so all of these functions are affected to some degree by drugs that act at dopamine receptors. It is likely that the catatonic symptoms seen in some schizophrenic patients, such as muscle stiffness, bizarre positions, and loss of spontaneous movement, are also due to disturbances in the dopamine system (Holden, 2003).

Norepinephrine (NE)

Areas of the brain where NE is found include the brain stem, cerebral cortex, limbic system, hypothalamus, cerebellum, and dorsal horn of the spinal cord. Processes that NE seems to influence include:

- state of arousal
- depressive disorders
- attention
- concentration
- regulation of blood pressure
- analgesia
- mania
- memory
- socialization

Serotonin (5-HT)

Serotonin is found mainly in the brain stem and in the neurons of the reticular formation. These reticular neurons project to many other areas of the brain. Serotonin is also found in the cortex, the

The Synapse

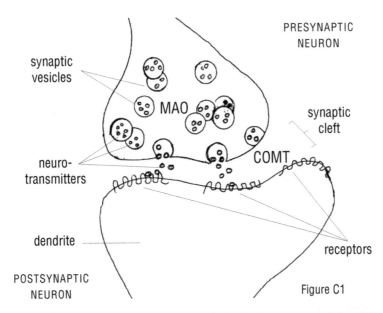

Figure C1

hypothalamus, the hippocampus, and the limbic system (Fig. B2) and has been shown to have a role in the processes of:

- depression
- falling asleep
- decreasing pain
- sexual activity
- regulating body temperature

In the depressive disorders, appetite, sexual desire and response, irritability, and impulse control are affected by decreased 5-HT.

NEUROPEPTIDE TRANSMITTERS

The number of neuropeptide transmitter substances exceeds the number of other transmitters in all categories. These peptides are found in some neurons that use amino acids and in some that use amines as neurotransmitters. In these neurons, there may be a release of two or more different transmitter substances, which allows for activation of more complex systems within the neuron (Bloom & Kupfer, 1995). Some neuropeptides that have been extensively investigated are vasopressin and oxytocin (both affect learning and memory), substance P, which is involved in transmission of painful stimuli, and opioid neuropeptides, which are involved in analgesic responses (see below) (DeVane, 2001).

Hypocretin (orexin)

This substance may be responsible for keeping us awake by preventing the spontaneous periods of REM that occur in narcolepsy. This neurotransmitter is present in low amounts in humans with narcolepsy, and is missing entirely in the dogs used as an animal model to study narcolepsy in the laboratory (Hungs & Miginot, 2001).

Opioid neuropeptides

Many areas of the central nervous system have high concentrations of specialized receptors called opioid receptors. These areas are the brain stem, medial thalamus, spinal cord, and limbic system, specifically the amygdala (see Fig. B2). Most of these areas are involved with the pain response. Some opioid receptors in the brain stem affect feelings of nausea and vomiting, others regulate blood pressure, stomach secretions, and the cough-response. Opioid-rich areas in the limbic system mediate emotional responses. The opioid neuropeptides in turn regulate dopamine levels (DeVane, 2001).

Substance P (neurokinin, NK)

Substance P is a type of neurokinin, a member of a group of neuropeptides called "tachykinins." Its receptor is called NK1. Neurokinin is a modulator which signals the intensity of noxious or aversive stimuli (nociception). Evidence suggests that substance P is also an integral part of central nervous system pathways involved in psychological stress (DeVane, 2001).

NK neurons are unique in that they have receptors all over the cell body. NK is found in both the brain and spinal cord. When an area is inflamed, both the amount of NK and the number of NK receptors increase. In the brain, NK receptors are found primarily in the limbic system, including two areas associated with emotional responses, the hypothalamus and the amygdala (see Fig. B2). Approximately 10% of all neurons in the amygdala are NK neurons. Stimulation of these neurons produces anxiety. The highest density of NK neurons is in the area of the thalamus known as the habenula (DeVane, 2001).

Neurokinins are present in neurons that are involved in the integration of pain, stress, and anxiety. NK1 is highly expressed in the hypothalamus, the pituitary, and the amygdala, brain regions that are critical for the regulation of emotions and neurochemical responses to stress (see Fig. B2). Also associated with the amygdala are neural pathways that respond to noxious or aversive stimuli (DeVane, 2001).

Although it makes logical sense, so far using NK antagonists to decrease pain has not been successful. The use of NK antagonists for treating anxiety disorders is being explored and a compound aprepitant/Emend, which is an NK antagonist, is now on the market to control nausea (Humphrey, 2003).

NEUROSTEROIDS

Neurosteroids have properties as neuromodulators of GABA, NMDA, and sigma receptors. Some neurosteroids are synthesized in the central nervous system and have a role in activation of glial cells (Belelli & Lambert, 2005; Bloom & Kupfer, 1995, Maurice et al., 1997).

NUCLEOTIDES

Nucleotides, such as adenosine triphosphate (ATP), sensitize neurons and enhance response to either amine or amino acid neurotransmitters. These compounds are sometimes called "third messengers."

Storage & Release of Monoamine Transmitters

NE, DA, and 5-HT are stored in synaptic vesicles; their release from vesicles is a calcium-dependent phenomenon. For release to take place after a nerve is stimulated, calcium must be present in the extracellular space. Transmitter release is dependent upon an influx of calcium ions (Ca^{+2}) into the nerve terminal. Medications known as "calcium channel blockers" inhibit Ca^{+2} influx and block neuronal firing (see Fig. A2).

Some mechanism must exist to terminate the action of transmitter substances. This can happen in various ways:

- After release, NE, DA, and 5-HT can be metabolized to inactive compounds by the enzyme which is present in the synapse, catechol-O-methyl transferase (COMT).
- Transmitter substances may be taken back into pre-synaptic nerve terminals (reuptake) and inactivated by the enzyme monoamine oxidase (MAO).
- After reuptake, they can be taken back into synaptic vesicles and stored for release at a later time.

References for Appendix C

Belelli, D. & Lambert, J. (2005). Neurosteroids: Endogenous regulators of the GABA receptor. *Nat. Rev. Neurosci.,* 6(7), 565–575.

Bloom, F. & Kupfer, D. (1995). *Psychopharmacology: The Fourth Generation of Progress.* New York: Raven Press.

DeVane, C. (2001). Substance P: A new era, a new role. *Pharmacotherapy,* 21(9), 1061–1069.

Gainetdinov, R., Wetsel, W., Jones, S., Levin, E., Jaber, M. & Caron, M. (1999). Role of serotonin in the paradoxical calming effect of psychostimulants on hyperactivity. *Science,* 283(5400), 397–401.

Gladwell, S. & Coote, J. (1999). Inhibitory and indirect excitatory effects of dopamine on sympathetic preganglionic neurons in the neonatal rat spinal cord in vitro. *Brain Research,* 818, 397–407.

Grundman, M. & Thai, L. (2000). Treatment of Alzheimer's disease: Rationale and strategies. *Neurol. Clin.,* 18(4), 807–828.

Holden, C. (2003). Excited by glutamate. *Science,* 20 June, (300), 1866–1868.

Humphrey, J. (2003). Medicinal chemistry of selective neurokinin-1 antagonists. *Current Topics in Medicinal Chemistry,* 3(12), 1423–435.

Hungs, M. & Mignot, E. (2001). Hypocretin/orexin, sleep and narcolepsy. *Bioessays,* 23, 397–408.

Johansen, C. (1992). *Psychopharmacology: Basic Mechanisms and Applied Interventions.* Washington, DC: APA.

Maurice, T., Junien, J. & Privat, A. (1997). Dehydroepiandrosterone sulfate attenuates dizocilpine-induced learning impairment in mice via sigma 1-receptors. *Behav. Brain Res.,* 83(1-2), 159–164.

Appendix D
Proposed Mechanisms of Action

As the workings of the central nervous system are better understood, the theories explaining the mechanisms of actions of the many drugs studied in psychopharmacology become more and more complex. The techniques and technologies required to investigate details of these processes in the CNS, and at the synapse in particular, are not yet available. For this reason, the specific, detailed mechanisms of action for most psychoactive substances are not yet completely clear.

Even when the primary effect of a drug is clear, this knowledge may not explain how the drug acts to create changes in emotions and behavior. This appendix presents proposed mechanisms of action for some of the drugs included in this book. The theories as to these mechanisms of action are constantly being refined and changed as new discoveries are made.

Many psychoactive substances affect the synthesis, storage, release, reuptake, or metabolism of the neuromodulators or neurotransmitters. The transmitter substances and their receptors have many subtypes and interact in complex and varied ways. Depending upon these actions in different parts of the brain, transmitters may have many different effects, stimulating neurons in one part of the brain and inhibiting them in another part.

By interfering in different ways with the transmission of information in the CNS, psychoactive compounds may enhance, mimic, or block the effects of transmitter substances. Transmitter substances interact with neurons containing other transmitter substances (2nd messengers or G-coupled proteins) which then go on to cause a cascade of events in the neuron which in the end leads to a change in emotional state or the growth or destruction of nerve cells.

Terms Used in the Study of Drugs

Comparisons of how drugs interact with receptors are frequently used to study and describe the properties of other drugs. It is important to understand the terms "agonist" and "antagonist," which are used when comparing a drug with unknown properties to a similar drug or transmitter substance that is already well-characterized.

Agonist: A drug or chemical compound that binds to the same receptor as the reference substance and exerts similar physiological and psychological effects.

Antagonist: A drug or chemical compound that displaces (competes) at the same receptor as the reference substance which leads to a decrease in physiological and psychological effects of the reference substance.

Partial agonist: A drug that has intermediate activity to the reference substance is termed a *partial agonist.*

Inverse agonist: A drug that has the opposite effect to the reference substance.

The Biogenic Amine Hypothesis

In the 1950s, researchers observed that reserpine, a drug used to treat hypertension, was causing depressive symptoms in about 15% of the patients taking it. It was hypothesized that taking reserpine leads to a depletion of NE and 5-HT in the CNS by first causing the release, and then preventing the reuptake, of these transmitters from the neuron's storage granules. When not inside storage granules, NE and 5-HT are broken down by the enzyme monoamine oxidase (MAO), leading to a depletion of NE and 5-HT. It was hypothesized that this depletion caused depression.

In 1965, as a result of these ideas, Joseph Schildkraut at Harvard posited the theory that clinical depression was associated with a deficiency of catecholamines (specifically NE) in certain brain regions and that mania was associated with an excess of NE. This developed into the biogenic amine hypothesis (Schildkraut, 1965).

The hypothesis is as follows: norepinephrine and serotonin are synthesized from the amino acids tyrosine and tryptophan, respectively. After the transmitters are synthesized, they are stored in the synaptic granules of the neuron, where they are protected from enzymatic degradation. When the nerve cell fires, NE or 5-HT is released from the storage granules into the cell's synaptic cleft; the NE or 5-HT then interacts with post-synaptic receptors. Depending upon appropriate stimulation or inhibition, the next neuron will either fire or be inhibited. At this point, the NE or 5-HT is either catabolized (broken down) by COMT at the synapse, or taken back up into the pre-synaptic side of the neuron and then catabolized by MAO. It was believed that antidepressant medications modified some part or parts of this process, causing some change in the neurotransmitter system leading to a change in mood (Schildkraut, 1965).

Present understanding

It is now known that this early hypothesis is an extremely simplified version of the complex chemistry of neurotransmission in the CNS. Since the 1960s, a wide variety of substances that act as neuromodulators and neurotransmitters have been, and continue to be, discovered. (See Appendix C). These compounds interact with various receptors that regulate the many functions and emotional states controlled in different parts of the CNS. The structure of the receptor is also much more complex than was initially imagined; every type of receptor can have a variety of different sites on it, with each site responding to different transmitter substances and drugs. Although current theories of how transmitters are synthesized, stored, released and affect emotions are much more detailed, complex and specific, they all have their origins in the biogenic amine theory.

Recent research has documented that the neurobiological substrate of depression, and the mechanism of action of antidepressants, are even more complex than just alterations at the synapse. Changes in the morphology of neurons, such as atrophy of neurons in the prefrontal cortex or the hypothalamus, or an increase in the number of CNS cortico-releasing factor (CRF) cell bodies, may all play a major role in the development of depression. It has also been hypothesized that changes caused by stress in the glucocorticoid receptors in certain regions of the brain (e.g., the hippocampus) contribute to the depressive symptoms (Bloom & Kupfer, 1995). (See Stress Hypothesis below.)

It is now clearer how the immune system contributes to the pathophysiology of depression. Some immune-mediated medical illnesses can lead to a behavioral syndrome similar to depression, and patients with a primary depressive illness will have alterations in their cytokine levels (the transmitters that are involved with the transmission of pain) (Dunn & Wang, 1995). The study of how these processes affect emotions and behavior is an extremely active area of research.

The Stress Hypothesis

Recently the stress hypothesis has been gaining credibility among brain researchers over the biogenic amine hypothesis. It posits that depression is caused when the brain's stress mechanism becomes overactive. When a person is stressed, the hypothalamus produces corticotropin-releasing hormone (CRH) which stimulates the pituitary gland, triggering the release of glucocorticoids (stress hormones such as cortisol) from the adrenal glands. The presence of these stress hormones may eventually lead to neuronal damage. If the stress is prolonged a shrinking of the hippocampus has been observed. This is a key site in the brain (see Fig. B2) for the action of antidepressant drugs (Adelson, 2005; Leonard, 2000).

This theory is supported by findings that the hippocampus is smaller in people who are chronically depressed (Leonard, 2000). Another supporting factor is the length of time it takes antidepressant medications to reach their optimal effect; this may indicate that neuronal growth is part of the recovery process (Leonard, 2000).

CHAPTER 1 (SLEEP & TREATMENT OF SLEEP DISORDERS)

Gamma-hydroxy butyrate/sodium oxybate

Although the specific mechanism of action of this drug remains unknown it has been demonstrated that gamma-hydroxybutyrate (GHB) binds to specific GHB receptors found only in the brain (Nishino, 2007). It also binds weakly to GABA receptors in the brain and in other tissues (Billard, et al., 2006). It is known that this binding to the GABA receptors induces the brain rhythms that are the basis of slow-wave (deep) sleep (Robinson, et al., 2007).

CHAPTER 2 (TREATMENT OF INSOMNIA & ANXIETY DISORDERS)

Sedative-hypnotic drugs/BzRAs

Most drugs in this class bind to the GABA receptor in a way that enhances the binding of GABA which leads to an inhibition of neuronal firing. There are different GABA receptor subtypes in different parts of the brain. It is believed that the binding to different subtypes is what causes the different effects (addictive potential, adverse effects) of drugs like the BzRAs. The z-compounds are structurally different from the BzRAs but they interact with the GABA receptor in the same way to enhance GABA binding. Since GABA is usually inhibitory, these compounds usually causes sedation.

Ramelteon

Ramelteon is the first compound with an entirely new mechanism of action to be approved as a sedative-hypnotic in 35 years. Ramelteon is a selective agonist for melatonin MT1 and MT2 receptor subtypes, which are most highly concentrated in the hypothalamic suprachiasmatic nucleus (SCN). The SCN functions as the master timekeeper of the circadian system. Melatonin agonist activity decreases the firing rate of SCN neurons, which decreases arousal and facilitates falling asleep (Neubauer, 2009).

Antihistamines for sleep induction

Antihistamines are believed to affect the histamine neurons that project from the hypothalamus to the cerebral cortex. When histamine neurons (which promote wakefulness) are blocked by an antihistamine this pathway is suppressed which leads to sedation. (Stahl, 2002).

CHAPTER 3 (ALCOHOL: USE & ABUSE)

The theorized mechanism of action for alcohol is complex and affects many different neurotransmitter systems and regions of the CNS. One factor that complicates understanding is that as alcohol concentration increases, its action in the brain becomes more diffuse and more parts of the brain are affected. Another complication is that the brain's response to alcohol is different depending on whether the exposure to alcohol is acute or chronic. Structural changes in the CNS are seen after chronic exposure to alcohol. Below is a simplified version of the current theory of how alcohol affects the CNS.

In general, ethanol modifies neural activity in the brain by modulating ion channels. (Ethanol activates G protein–gated K+ channels, but the molecular mechanism is not well understood.)

Specifically:

1. Alcohol has specific effects on GABA and glutamate receptors (Bonner, 1994; Tabakoff & Hoffman, 1993).

2. GABA and glutamate are responsible for much of the inhibitory and excitatory activity in the CNS.

   a) At first, alcohol increases the inhibitory action of GABA receptors and decreases the excitatory activity of glutamate receptors.

   b) Enhancement of GABA activity is responsible for the sedating effect of alcohol.

   c) Decrease in glutamate activity in the hippocampus may be the reason for the decreased ability to form new memories while intoxicated (Kuhn, et al., 1998).

   d) The inhibiting effect on the hippocampus accounts for

lapses in memory, or in severe instances, blackouts.

e) Chronic ingestion of alcohol can lead to cell injury and death by making neurons more sensitive to excititoxicity produced by glutamate (Tabakoff & Hoffman, 1993).

3. Alcohol ingestion causes increased release of DA in reward centers of the brain (Tabakoff & Hoffman, 1993).

a) DA release is probably mediated by GABA neurons that connect to DA neurons in reward centers of the brain, leading to the experience of pleasure.

b) The increase in DA activity only takes place while the alcohol level in the blood is rising, not when the level is constant or falling. Because of this, the drinker in search of this pleasurable experience may be motivated to continue drinking to keep the blood-alcohol level rising (Kuhn, et al., 1998).

There is some evidence suggesting a common pathway for the mechanism of action of opioids and alcohol. Acute use of alcohol leads to increased endorphin levels. Opioid receptors in the CNS react differentially to the acute or chronic presence of alcohol. This contributes to the differences in mood seen when people who are habituated to alcohol drink when compared with the response of people who are not habituated (Bonner, 1994).

Acamprosate

Acamprosate is believed to reduce the overaction of the glutamate NMDA system seen with chronic alcohol exposure. It may act by reducing both the release of glutamate from the presynaptic nerve terminal and by reducing over-activation due to up-regulated postsynaptic NMDA receptors (Littleton & Zieglgansberger, 2003).

Disulfiram

Disulfiram/Antabuse inhibits the enzymatic oxidation of acetaldehyde to acetic acid during the metabolism of alcohol to carbon dioxide (CO_2) and water (H_2O). The inhibition of enzyme activity caused by disulfiram is irreversible (until more enzyme is synthesized).

This blockage of enzymatic activity leads to a buildup of acetaldehyde. Drinking while taking disulfiram results in a buildup of acetaldehyde and produces unpleasant (and possibly toxic) effects. The chemical reaction that illustrates the action of disulfiram can be seen below:

alcohol ⟶ acetaldehyde ⟶ acetic acid ⟶ carbon dioxide + water

Figure D1

disulfiram blocks here

Naltrexone

Naltrexone/Revia acts as an antagonist at the opioid receptor. Through this function it is believed to modulate the dopamine reward pathway. This leads to a reduction both in the frequency of drinking and the number of drinks consumed per day (Anton & Swift, 2003).

CHAPTER 4 (TREATMENT OF DEPRESSIVE DISORDERS)

Selective serotonin reuptake inhibitors (SSRIs)

As the name indicates, these drugs prevent the reuptake of 5-HT into the presynaptic space by binding to the 5-HT reuptake transporter molecule so the 5-HT remains in the synaptic cleft longer.

There may be a lag time of several weeks before maximal decrease of depressive symptoms is experienced. The reason for the lag is not clear; there is some indication that this may be due to the time it takes for neurons to grow. Although called SSRIs, these drugs also have some affect on NE and, to lesser extent, DA (Lane & Baldwin, 1995).

Tricyclic & heterocyclic antidepressants (TCAs & HCAs)

Tricyclic and heterocyclic antidepressants act by interfering with the transport of NE and 5-HT back into the presynaptic side of the synaptic cleft (in the same way as the SSRIs do, by binding to the transporter molecule), resulting in an increase in NE and 5-HT in the synaptic cleft.

Monoamine oxidase inhibitors (MAOIs)

The MAOIs bind to MAO (an enzyme which normally breaks down the monoamines NE, 5-HT, and DA) thus inactivating the MAO, resulting in higher levels of these neuromodulators. The decreased breakdown of NE and 5-HT results in a decrease of the symptoms of depression.

L-tryptophan and 5-HTP

Other substances that lead to an increase in 5-HT and NE at the synapse may alleviate symptoms of depression. Taking l-tryptophan or 5-HTP (both of which are precursors to 5-HT) will enhance the effect of antidepressant medications. For some people these are effective as antidepressants when taken by themselves (Shaw, et al., 2002).

CHAPTER 5 (TREATMENT OF BIPOLAR DISORDER)

Lithium

Even though there have been millions of prescriptions written for lithium over the last 60 years, researchers are still not certain as to how it exerts its effects. Here are some of the theories being investigated:

Lithium may promote neuron growth in brain tissue by depressing a mechanism that normally prevents neurons from growing. This allows neurons to form new connections and grow into unoccupied spaces. Lithium may also increase levels of brain-derived neurotrophic factor (BDNF), which has been shown to stimulate neuronal growth (Medina, 2003).

It has been observed that cells exposed to lithium for a week are protected from over-stimulation and death that can be caused by the presence of large amounts of glutamate (Nonaka, et al., 1998). Researchers have demonstrated that lithium can both slow down and speed up the glutamate reuptake system (which leads to a stabilization of glutamate levels). Lithium may exert its effect by limiting the influx of calcium into nerve cells (which usually takes place in the presence of glutamate and leads to cell death) (Nonaka, et al., 1998).

If this hypothesis is correct, then taking lithium may also be helpful in other situations where there is cell death, such as with a cardiovascular accident (stroke), and with Parkinson's, Alzheimer's, and Huntington's diseases (Dixon & Hokin, 1988).

Anticonvulsant medications

Most anticonvulsant medications have widespread effects in the CNS. They affect neuronal transmission in the limbic system, which leads to their anticonvulsant properties. Anticonvulsant medications are believed to act through a variety of mechanisms, including through SV2A (synaptic vesicle protein), voltage-gated potassium channels, ionotropic and metabotropic glutamate receptors, and gap junctions. Some act as agonists at GABA receptors in the CNS, resulting in neuronal inhibition and therefore a lessening of convulsions (Pope, et al., 1991).

Chapter 6 (Stimulants: Use & Abuse)

Amphetamines

Amphetamines are known to lead to a decrease in the transport of NE and DA back into the presynaptic terminal by binding to the DA transporter molecule. They also inhibit the enzyme MAO. This leads to an increased amount of NE and DA at the synapse. The increased DA at the synapse may be the cause of the paranoid psychosis sometimes seen in chronic amphetamine users. DA has a role in the reward system in the CNS. All processes of addiction have some connection to the DA system (Fleckenstein, et al., 2007: Schuckit, 1997).

Drugs for attention deficit disorders

The reason stimulant drugs have a calming effect in people with ADHD is not well-understood. It seems clear that NE has a role in the effects, and it is believed that 5-HT also is involved in the action of the drugs used for this purpose. Recent research suggests involvement of NE and DA transporter mechanisms (Gainetdinov, et al., 1999; MacMaster, et al., 2002).

Cocaine

Taking cocaine leads to a decrease in the reuptake of NE and DA from the synapse. It has been demonstrated that cocaine strongly binds to the DA reuptake transporter molecule; this prevents reuptake of DA into the presynaptic cells, leading to an increased DA effect at the synapse (Schuckit, 1997). Large amounts of DA at the synapse leads to the characteristic euphoria and stimulation (rush) experienced when cocaine is used. The neurons that are stimulated by DA in the reward centers of the brain then stimulate distant neurons to release endogenous opioids and GABA (Dackis, 2007).

Nicotine

Research has shown that nornicotine (a major alkaloid found in tobacco and an active metabolite of nicotine) increases DA release in the CNS. The nornicotine stimulates nicotinic receptors in the CNS (acting as an agonist at these receptors), which then causes the release of DA and the rewarding effects of nicotine (Teng, et al., 1997).

Varenicline tartrate

Varenicline/Chantix is an nicotinic receptor partial agonist. It is believed to work by counteracting the decrease in DA levels during withdrawal and by blocking the stimulating and dopamine-releasing effects when nicotine is consumed (Naiura, et al., 2006)

Caffeine

Caffeine is believed to act as a nonselective antagonist of adenosine (an inhibitory neurotransmitter) receptors (Kaplan, et al., 1992). The caffeine molecule is structurally similar to adenosine and binds to adenosine receptors on the surface of cells without activating them.

Adenosine, because it plays a role in fundamental (ATP-related) energy metabolism, is found in every part of the body, but it has special functions in the brain. There is a great deal of evidence that concentrations of brain adenosine are increased by various types of metabolic stress including anoxia (lack of oxygen) and ischemia (lack of blood). Evidence also indicates that brain adenosine acts to protect the brain by suppressing neural activity and by increasing blood flow through receptors located on vascular smooth muscle. By counteracting adenosine, caffeine reduces resting cerebral blood flow between 22% and 30% (Addicott, et al., 2009). This may be the reason caffeine is helpful in headache treatment. Caffeine is also known to affect ACh in the cortex, which may be linked to caffeine's ability to increase mental acuity (Acquas, et al., 2002).

CHAPTER 7 (TREATMENT OF PSYCHOTIC DISORDERS)

Antipsychotic drugs

The SGAs have been more extensively studied than the FGAs because of the advanced research techniques now available. All antipsychotic drugs (first and second generation) influence the response of the CNS to NE, DA, and 5-HT to varying degrees and in various areas of the brain. These neuromodulators and their receptors have many subtypes which are active in different parts of the brain and have different effects. The areas of the CNS which are most affected by these medications are the:

- hypothalamus
- basal ganglia
- limbic system
- cerebral cortex

Second generation antipsychotic medications (SGAs)

The SGAs affect 5-HT transmission to a greater extent than do the FGAs. In addition to their effects on dopamine, some SGAs also affect transmission at histamine, GABA, glutamate, NMDA, and ACh sites. Studies have shown a relationship between DA and GABA. As DA levels increase, GABA levels decrease. Low levels of GABA are correlated with disorganized thought processes. High levels of DA may suppress GABA, resulting in a thought disorder. The inhibition of neuronal activity due to GABA may be necessary to keep the number of signals in the CNS at a level and frequency that can be received and assimilated in a way that makes sense (Acquas, et al., 2002).

Dopamine system stabilizers (DSSs)

The DSSs act as partial DA agonists (Tandon, 2002). They increase DA transmission in some parts of the brain (frontal lobes) where it is believed DA is too low; this increase helps with the negative symptoms of schizophrenia. DSSs decrease DA transmission in other parts of the CNS (limbic system) where it is thought the DA levels are too high; this decrease helps alleviate the positive symptoms of schizophrenia (Stahl, 2001).

CHAPTER 8 (PAIN & TREATMENTS OF PAIN)

Pain medications

One way opioids exert their effect is by inhibiting neuronal activity by selectively binding to specific, opioid receptors in the CNS. Many of these sites are in the hypothalamus. Large numbers of opioid receptors are also found outside the CNS. They are abundant in the intestine, where opioids act as antidiarrhea agents by slowing peristalsis. The compound paregoric acts in this way and is often given to children with severe diarrhea. Opioids also act as neuromodulators and inhibit the release of substance P, DA, and ACh, all leading to a decrease in the transmission of the pain impulse (Mantyh, 2000).

Nonsteroidal anti-inflammatory agents (NSAIDs)

One site where NSAIDs are believed to act is at the glycine receptors in the spinal cord. Normally, prostaglandins inhibit glycine transmission, allowing pain signals to be transmitted to the brain from the spinal cord. NSAIDs block prostaglandin production, which leads to a decrease in pain signals going to the brain (Marx, 2004).

Morphine & the endorphins

Morphine and related compounds exert their analgesic and other actions by interacting with specific opioid receptors. The specificity of these receptors led investigators to postulate the existence of an endogenous (internally generated) substance in the CNS that is analogous to the opioids. These endogenous substances were found and named endorphins, for "endogenous morphine-like substances." The first endorphins to be characterized were named enkephalins; these were found to be only mildly analgesic, but to have a high addictive potential. It is believed that enkephalins act as inhibitory neurotransmitters. Chronic use of opioids leads to a decrease in the production of endogenous enkephalins and endorphins.

The opioid receptors, which were previously called delta, kappa, and mu, have been reclassified by a subcommittee of the International Union of Pharmacology as OP1 (delta), OP2 (kappa), and OP3 (mu). Their different properties are:

OP1 receptors: These mediate analgesia, sedation, and possibly the release of some hormones.

OP2 receptors: These are responsible for analgesia, dysphoria and some psychotomimetic effects (e.g., disorientation and/or depersonalization), and sedation.

OP3 receptors: These are responsible for analgesia, euphoria, respiratory depression, and meiosis (a type of cell division).

Methadone

Methadone, like most of the commonly used opioids (oxycodone, fentanyl, hydrocodone), is an opioid receptor agonist and consequently reduces pain. A second mechanism by which methadone provides analgesia is by acting as an (NMDA) receptor antagonist (Davis & Inturrisi, 1999).

Naltrexone

Naltrexone is a competitive antagonist at the opioid receptor, effectively blocking the nerve cell's ability to bind to endorphins and opioids. When naltrexone is present one cannot experience the pleasureable sensations induced by opioids. Naltrexone will cause withdrawal if taken by someone who is physically dependent on opioids (Shader, 2003).

Buprenorphine

This drug acts on OP3 receptors to cause analgesia, euphoria, and other opioid effects. It is a partial agonist to diacetylmorphine/heroin, but less potent. It binds strongly to the OP3 receptor, preventing euphoria if other opioids are used. It is long-acting, which makes the detox process more gentle. For those who have been heavy drug users, it can trigger withdrawal symptoms (Fingerhood, et al., 2001).

Chapter 9 (Consciousness-Alerting Drugs)

Dimethyltryptamine (DMT) & ayahuasca

DMT, either by itself or in ayahuasca, exerts its effects by acting as an antagonist at 5-HT receptors (Pierce & Petroutka, 1989). Ayahuasca also contains an MAO inhibitor which, by preventing enzymatic degradation by MAO, allows for absorption of the DMT and prolongs its activity (Calloway, et al., 1999).

Lysergic acid diethylamide (LSD, "acid")

Lysergic acid/LSD is in a group of compounds called the indolealkylamines. Because it resembles 5-HT in chemical structure, it may act as a 5-HT agonist. It also has some effect at the NE receptors. The specific mechanism of action of LSD remains unclear.

Tetrahydrocannabinol (THC)

Analogous to the cannabinoids found in marijuana and hashish, there are endogenous substances called endocannabinoids (e.g., anandamide) found in the CNS. These bind to specific cannabinoid receptors, and act as retrograde messengers (the endocannabinoids bind to presynaptic receptors) in the brain. Synthesis and release of the endocannabinoids is due to postsynaptic depolarization. Inactivation of the endocannabinoids is probably due to an enzyme that specifically degrades this class of lipids (fats) (Bracey, et al., 2002).

Recent research indicates that the endogenous cannabinoid system (which is also activated by the THC in marijuana) protects neurons against cell death after brain trauma (Mechoulam & Lichtman, 2003). The exact function (or functions) of the endocannabinoids, or how they relate to the THC in marijuana, is not yet understood.

MDMA ("ecstasy")

MDMA causes both the release of and a decrease in the reuptake of 5-HT. It also binds to the receptors for other neurotransmitters, leading to specific effects (e.g., hallucinations, hypertension). It is thought that DA is involved in the pleasurable effects of MDMA (Solowij, 1993).

Phencyclidine (PCP) & Ketamine

PCP and ketamine block (act as antagonists) at the N-methyl-D-aspartate (NMDA) receptors. This blocking of the receptors is believed to cause analgesia by reducing the capacity of neuronal projections to conduct and coordinate signals. Phencyclidine and ketamine may cause cell death in some neurons (Jansen, 1996).

Phencyclidine is known to induce psychotic episodes in normal subjects, and to exacerbate psychosis in schizophrenics. Phencyclidine and ketamine appear to enhance glutamate transmission at non-NMDA receptors. This may lead to a disorganization of cortical activity (as is found in schizophrenia) (Moghaddam, 2003; O'Donnell & Grace, 1998). The brain regions that appear to play a role in the pathophysiology of schizophrenia (prefrontal cortex, hippocampus, basal ganglia) are the areas most likely involved in the consciousness altering action of phencyclidine (Jansen, 1996; O'Donnell & Grace, 1998).

Peyote

As with most botanicals, there are many chemical compounds present in the cactus *Lophophora williamsii* that might cause the symptoms of intoxication. There are 32 alkaloids in peyote, most of which are in the phenylethylamine category; many of these may have psychedelic effects. The most widely studied is mescaline, which resembles DA, NE, and the amphetamines in its chemical structure. The specific mechanism of action remains unclear.

Psilocybin

The active ingredient in psilocybin is 4, hydroxymethyltryptamine. This molecule is similar to 5-HT and tryptophan (a 5-HT precursor).

Because of this similarity, it is believed to act at the serotonin receptors (Vollenweider, et al., 1999).

CHAPTER 10 (COGNITION-ENHANCING DRUGS)

Cholinergic drugs

These drugs affect the ACh system in the CNS and seem to work in conjunction with the steroid hormones. It has been demonstrated that when the adrenal glands have been removed, cholinergic drugs have no effect. ACh levels decrease with age. This decrease may be one factor that leads to the loss of cognitive functioning which is often seen with aging. Anticholinergic drugs act synergistically when taken in combination with other nootropics (Moghaddam, 2003).

Ampakines

The group of drugs called ampakines activate AMPA-type receptors. Through this activation they enhance glutamate transmission in the CNS. It is believed that this enhancement may help to improve cognitive abilities (Berry-Kravis, et al., 2002).

References for Appendix D

Acquas, E., Gianluigi, T. & Di Chiara, G. (2002). Differential effects of caffeine on dopamine and acetylcholine transmission in brain areas of drug-naive and caffeine-pretreated rats. *Neuropsychopharm.*, 27, 182–193.

Adelson, R. (2005). Hard-hitting hormones: The stress-depression link. *Monitor on Psychology*, Jan., 24-25.

Addicott, M., Yang, L., Peiffer, A., Burnett, L., Burdette, J., Chen, M., Hayasaka, S., Kraft, R., Maldjian, J. & Laurienti, P. (2009). The effect of daily caffeine use on cerebral blood flow: How much caffeine can we tolerate? *Hum. Brain Mapp.*, 30(10), 3102–114.

Anton, R. & Swift, R. (2003). Current pharmacotherapies of alcoholism: A U.S. perspective. *Am. J. Addict.*, 12(Suppl. 1), S53-S68.

Berry-Kravis, E., Hagerman, R. & Cook E. (2002). New drug that enhances glutamate transmission in the brain being evaluated for Fragile X. *Science Daily Magazine*. Retrieved October 22, 2003 from http://www.rush.edu/

Billard, M., Bassetti, C. & Dauvilliers, Y. (2006). EFNS guidelines on the management of narcolepsy. *Eur. J. Neurol.*, 13(10), 1035-048.

Bloom, F. & Kupfer, D. (Eds.) (1995). *Psychopharmacology: The Fourth Generation of Progress*. New York: Raven Press.

Bonner, A. (1994). Biological mechanisms of alcohol dependence. *Current Opinion in Psychiatry*, 7, 262–268.

Bracey, M., Hanson, M., Masuda, K., Stevens, R. & Cravatt, B. (2002). Structural adaptations in a membrane enzyme that terminates endocannabinoid signaling. *Science*, 298, 1793–1796.

Callaway, J., McKenna, D., Grob, C., Brito, G., Raymon, L., Poland, R., Andrade, E., Andrade, E. & Mash, D. (1999). Pharmacokinetics of hoasca alkaloids in healthy humans. *J. Ethnopharmacol.*, 65, 243–256.

Dackis, C. (2007). The neurobiology of cocaine dependence and its clinical implications. *Psychiatric Times*, March, 62-66, 67.

Daly, J. & Fredholm, B. (1998). Caffeine-an atypical drug of dependence. *Drug and Alcohol Dependence*, 51, 199–206.

Davis, A. & Inturrisi, C. (1999). d-Methadone blocks morphine tolerance and N-methyl-d-aspartate-induced hyperalgesia. *J. Pharmacology and Experimental Therapeutics*, 289(2), 1048-053.

Dixon, J. & Hokin, L. (1988). Lithium acutely inhibits and chronically up-regulates and stabilizes glutamate uptake by presynaptic nerve endings in mouse cerebral cortex. *Proceedings of the National Academy of Sciences*, July 7, 95(14), 8363–8368.

Dunn, A. & Wang, J. (1995). Cytokine effects on CNS biogenic amines. *Neuroimmunomodulation*, 2, 319.

Fingerhood, M., Thompson, M. & Jasinski, D. (2001). A comparison of clonidine and buprenorphine in the outpatient treatment of opiate withdrawal. *Substance Abuse*, 22(3), 193–199.

Fleckenstein, A., Volz, T., Riddle, E., Gibb, J. &. Hanson, G. (2007). New insights into the mechanism of action of amphetamines. *Annual Review of Pharmacology and Toxicology*, 47, 681-698.

Gainetdinov, R., Wetsel, W., Jones, S, Levin, E., Jaber, M. & Caron, M. (1999). Role of serotonin in the paradoxical calming effect of psychostimulants on hyperactivity. *Science*, 283(5400), 397–401.

Jansen, K. (1996) Using ketamine to induce the near-death experience: Mechanism of action and therapeutic potential. *Yearbook for Ethnomedicine and the Study of Consciousness* (Jahrbuch fur Ethnomedizin und Bewubtseinsforschung), Issue 4, 1995, 55–81. Ratsch, C. & Baker, J. (Eds.), VWB, Berlin.

Kaplan, G. Greenblatt, D., Kent, M., Cotreau, M., Arcelin, G. & Shader, R. (1992). Caffeine-induced behavioral stimulation is dose-dependent and associated with A1 adenosine receptor occupancy. *Neuropsychopharm.*, 6, 145–153.

Kuhn, C., Schwartzwelder, S. & Wilson, W. (1998). *BUZZED: The Straight Facts About the Most Used and Abused Drugs from Alcohol to Ecstasy.* New York: W. W. Norton and Co.

Lane, R., Baldwin, D. & Preskorn, S. (1995). The SSRIs: Advantages, disadvantages and differences. *J Psychopharmacol.*, 9(Suppl.), 163–178.

Leonard, B. (2000). Stress, depression and the activation of the immune system. *World J. Biol. Psychiatry*, 1(1), 17–25.

Littleton, J. & Zieglgansberger, W. (2003). Pharmacological mechanisms of naltrexone and acamprosate in the prevention of relapse in alcohol dependence. *Am. J. Addict.*, 12(Suppl. 1), S3-S11.

MacMaster, F., Carrey, N., Sparkes, S. & Kusumakar, V. (2002). Proton spectroscopy in medication-free pediatric attention deficit/hyperactivity disorder: A preliminary case series. *J. Child Adolescent Psychopharm.*, Winter, 12, 331–336.

Mantyh, P. (2000). Understanding substance P and the substance P receptor. Presented at the XXIInd Congress of the Collegium Internationale Neuro-Psychopharmacologicum (CINP); July 10, Brussels, Belgium. Abstract.

Marx, J. (2004). Locating a new step in pain's pathway. *Science,* 304, 811.

Mechoulam, R. & Lichtman, A. (2003). Stout guards of the central nervous system. *Science,* 302(5642), 65–67.

Medina, J. (2003). Intracellular signaling and mood stabilizers. *Psychiatric Times,* XX(12), 32–36.

Moghaddam, B. (2003). Glutamate and disorders of cognition and motivation, April 13–15, *New York Academy of Sciences.*

Naiura, R., Jones, C. & Kirkpatrick, P. (2006). Fresh from the pipeline: Varenicline. *Nature Reviews Drug Discovery,* 5, 537-538.

Neubauer, D. (2009). Insomnia: Recent advances in pharmacological management. Retrieved March 22, 2010. http://www.psychiatrictimes.com/sleep disorders/content/article/1145628/1490698

Nishino, S. (2007). Clinical and neurobiological aspects of narcolepsy. *Sleep Med.,* 8(4), 373-399.

Nonaka, S., Hough, C. & Chuang, D. (1998). Chronic lithium treatment robustly protects neurons in the central nervous system against excitotoxicity by inhibiting N-methyl-D-aspartate receptor-mediated calcium influx. *Proceedings of the National Academy of Sciences,* March 3, 95, 2641–2647.

O'Donnell, P. & Grace, A. (1998). Phencyclidine interferes with the hippocampal gating of nucleus accumbens neuronal activity in vivo. *Neuroscience,* 87(4), 823–830.

Pierce, P. & Peroutka, S. (1989). Hallucinogenic drug interactions with neurotransmitter receptor binding sites in human cortex. *Psychopharm.,* 97, 118–122.

Pope, H., Mc Elroy, S., Keck, P. & Hudson, J. (1991). Valproate in the treatment of acute mania: A placebo controlled study. *Arch. Gen. Psychiatry,* 48, 62–68.

Robinson, D. & Keating, G. (2006). Sodium oxybate: A review in its use in the management of narcolepsy. *CNS Drugs,* 21(4), 337-354.

Schildkraut, J. (1965). The catecholamine hypothesis of affective disorders: A review of supporting evidence. *Am. J. Psychiatry,* 122, 509.

Schuckit, M. (1997). Science, medicine, and the future: Substance use disorders. *BMJ,* 314, 1605–1608.

Shader, R. (2003). Antagonists, inverse agonists, and protagonists. *J. Clinical Psychopharmacol.,* 23(4), 321–322.

Shaw, K., Turner, J. & Del Mar, C. (2002). Tryptophan and 5-hydroxytryptophan for depression. *Cochrane Database Syst. Rev.,* (1):CD003198.

Solowij, N. (1993). Ecstasy (3,4-methylenedioxymethamphetamine). *Current Opinion in Psychiatry,* 6, 411–415.

Stahl, S. (2001). Dopamine system stabilizers, aripiprazole, and the next generation of antipsychotics, Part I: "Goldilocks" actions at dopamine receptors, and Part II: Illustrating their mechanisms of action. *J. Clinical Psychiatry*, 62(11), 841–842 and 62(12), 923–924.

Stahl, S. (2002). Awakening to the psychopharmacology of sleep and arousal: Novel neurotransmitters and wake-promoting drugs. *J. Clinical Psychiatry*, 63(4), 339–402.

Tabakoff, B. & Hoffman, P. (1993). The neurochemistry of alcohol. *Current Opinion in Psychiatry*, 6, 388–394.

Tandon, R. (2002). New steps in the evolution of antipsychotics: The role of partial agonists. *U.S. Psych. Congress*, October, Las Vegas, NV.

Teng, L., Crooks, P., Buckston, S. & Dwoskin, L. (1997). Nicotinic-receptor mediation of S(-)nornicotine-evoked [^{3}H] overflow from rat striatal slices preloaded with [^{3}H] dopamine. *Psychopharm. Exp. Ther.*, 283(2), 778–787.

Vollenweider, F., Vontobel, P., Hell, D. & Leenders, K. (1999). 5-HT modulation of dopamine release in basal ganglia in psilocybin-induced psychosis in man— A PET study with [^{11}C] raclopride. *Neuropsychopharm.*, 20(5), 424–433.

Appendix E

Other Types of Drug Responses

TOLERANCE

In pharmacological terms, "tolerance" means a decreased response to a drug; an increased dosage is then necessary to obtain the desired effect. Tolerances to different effects of a drug develop at different rates. For example, a particular sedative may have a number of effects. It may induce sleep, cause euphoria, and inhibit psychomotor performance. Since tolerance to the psychomotor effect develops more slowly than tolerance to the euphoric effect, a person might increase the dosage of the sedative drug to obtain a desired amount of euphoria while not realizing that this increase may, due to different amounts of tolerance, result in a dangerous impairment of the ability to drive.

TYPES OF TOLERANCE

Enzymatic or dispositional tolerance

This type of tolerance is due to an increase in the rate of production of liver enzymes that are synthesized to metabolize a drug. This leads to an increased rate of drug metabolism. The more rapid metabolism can lead to taking higher doses of the drug to maintain a desired level of effect.

Cellular or pharmacodynamic tolerance

This type of tolerance occurs when the target cell or receptor for the drug changes over time due to exposure to the drug. When this occurs, a higher dose is required to produce a desired effect. An example is the phenomenon known as "down-regulation" of receptors.

Cross-tolerance

This is a type of cellular tolerance that occurs when tolerance develops to drugs in the same class, or in similar classes, due to a change in the receptor for those drugs. An example is the cross-tolerance that develops between opioids and other types of narcotics. A person taking one type of pain killer may develop a tolerance to others even when the drugs are completely different in their chemical structures. Some cross-tolerance can even develop between drugs in different classes (e.g. between alcohol and sedatives).

> **Note: Any drug may cause the development of any or all of the different types of tolerances.**

PHYSICAL DEPENDENCE, ADDICTION, & ABUSE

Physical dependence

Physical dependence has been defined in many different ways. One definition states that physical dependence occurs when a person who has been taking a particular drug on a regular basis begins to require that drug to function normally, experiences withdrawal symptoms with abstinence, and is able to terminate the withdrawal symptoms by taking the drug. It is sometimes difficult to clearly delineate between physical and psychological symptoms of withdrawal (e.g., anxiety symptoms that occur with withdrawal from marijuana).

The *DSM* states that dependence involves the impaired control of psychoactive substance use, and continued use despite adverse consequences. It includes legal, illegal, and prescription drugs on its list of drugs that have a potential for substance dependence. Alcohol, amphetamines, antianxiety drugs, cannabis, cocaine, hallucinogens, nicotine, and sedatives are a few of the drugs of potential abuse listed in the *DSM*. It is mainly the adverse consequences with use of a drug or substance that define abuse or addiction.

In this book the term "physical dependence" is used to denote a state of physiological need for a drug. In other words, if the drug is not taken, physical withdrawal symptoms will be experienced. Physical dependence is not meant to signify that a drug is being used in an addictive or abusive manner.

Addiction

In this book, the term "addiction" is used when taking a drug leads to some destructive consequence in a person's life. The amount or frequency of drug-use is not the determining factor. For example, someone can be a binge drinker and consume alcohol only once a year, but if there are negative consequences to that drinking episode the use is considered an addiction.

Abuse

The term "abuse" in the *DSM* indicates maladaptive patterns of psychoactive substance use. This category includes substance use in situations that may be physically hazardous, such as while driving. It also includes continued use despite knowledge that a social, psychological, occupational, or physical problem is being caused by use of the psychoactive substance. According to the *DSM*, the symptoms must have persisted for at least one month.

WITHDRAWAL

Withdrawal is a syndrome of autonomic dysfunction that occurs when someone who is physically dependent on a drug stops taking it. Withdrawal symptoms may or may not be the same as those of the original disorder for which the medication was taken. For many drugs, withdrawal symptoms are the opposite of the drug's effects. For example, if a drug is taken to decrease anxiety (typically a BzRA), anxiety and agitation will increase when the drug is withdrawn.

ALLERGIC REACTIONS

Another common type of response to a drug is an allergic reaction. This type of reaction involves the immune system. One person's immune system may react violently to a substance or drug that is harmless to the general population. Specifically, in an allergic reaction an antibody (usually immunoglobulin E) will bind to an allergen (the drug) and to a mast cell containing heparin (an anticoagulant) and histamine, or to a basophil (a type of white blood cell). This process initiates a release of histamine and other chemicals into the bloodstream. The release of these substances causes swelling, heat, and itching.

A classical allergic reaction is defined very specifically. This type of reaction is very serious and can be fatal. Often, the first sign of an allergic reaction is the development of a skin rash. If a rash develops while someone is taking medication, the prescribing physician should be notified immediately. It is likely that the physician will advise that the drug be discontinued and never taken again. The physician must be informed by the client of any drug allergies. Many drugs are chemically similar, and an allergy to one drug may serve as a warning of a possible allergic reaction to others in the same chemical class.

Allergies, intolerances, & sensitivities

The term "allergy" is now being used more broadly to include what in the past had been called the "intolerances" or "sensitivities" that some people have to milk, wheat, or other foods. Digestive problems and headaches are the usual symptoms seen with these food intolerances or sensitivities. One cause can be an absence of the enzyme necessary to digest the specific food properly (e.g., with lactose intolerance the enzyme lactase, which digests milk products, may be either present in small amounts, or missing entirely).

It is also possible for a person to have a true allergic reaction to a food or a food group. Well-known examples of this are allergies to shellfish or peanuts. The symptoms of this type of food allergy usually include burning of the lips or mouth, skin rash, severe cramping, and diarrhea. If a food allergy is suspected, one should not consume the suspect food and consult a physician. This type of classical allergy can be fatal.

PLACEBO EFFECTS

A placebo is defined as a substance that contains no known pharmacologically-active ingredient, yet elicits a therapeutic response.

The specific mechanism for this type of response is not yet understood, but it is thought to be due mainly to the patient's expectations. The standard finding is that a placebo is effective in about 33% of the people to whom it is administered. When new drugs are developed, it is important to keep in mind that usually a response rate much higher than the response to a placebo needs to occur for the drug to be considered pharmacologically active.

This standard for therapeutic effectiveness is influenced by many factors, including the seriousness of the disease the drug is designed to treat, the potential adverse effects or lack of adverse effects from the drug, and the availability of alternative treatments or medications.

Final Thoughts

New psychoactive medications are constantly being developed. It is neither practical, nor necessary, for the psychotherapist to study the mechanisms of actions of these drugs or learn details such as which neurotransmitters are affected, or memorize the specific doses of all the medications. If a client is taking medication, what is important is that the therapist know the class of drug being taken and recognize whether the drug is an appropriate treatment for the presenting symptoms.

It is also vital that the therapist be able to assess whether a client might benefit from the use of psychoactive medication, be able to discuss the use of psychoactive medication in a knowledgeable and unbiased way, and work collegially with the psychiatrist or other medical professional who is prescribing the medication. With the increased use of psychoactive medications, these skills have become important prerequisites for all psychotherapists.

Common Psychiatric Medications & Nonprescription Drugs

Sedative-Hypnotic & Antianxiety Medications

Generic name/Brand name®	Avg. daily dose (mg)
Benzodiazepines (BzRAs)	
alprazolam/Xanax	0.25–8
chlordiazepoxide/Librium	5–250
clonazepam/Klonopin	1–6
diazepam/Valium	2–40
flurazepam/Dalmane	15–60
lorazepam/Ativan	0.5–1
triazolam/Halcion	0.25–0.5
temazepam/Restoril	15–30
z-compounds	
escataloprm/Lunesta	1–3
zaleplon/Sonata	5–20
zolpidem/Ambien/Ambien/ CR/Edluar(sublingual)	5–10
Atypical Hypnotics	
ramelteon/Rozerem	8
Other Medications for Anxiety	
atenolol/Tenormin	25–100
buspirone/Buspar	15–60
clonidine/Catapres	0.1–3
escitalopram/Lexapro	10
hydroxyzine/Atarax/Vistaril	50–400
propranolol/Inderal	80–640

Many SSRI antidepressants are now used as a first-line treatment for anxiety.

Opioids & Pain Medications

buprenorphine/Buprenex/Subutex	16
buprenorphine + naloxone/Suboxone	4–24
codeine	45–240
fentanyl/Actiq (transmucosal)/ Duragesic/Sublimaze (transdermal)	varies
hydrocodone/Vicodin/Lortab	7.5–30
hydromorphone/Dilaudid	1 & up
meperidine/Demerol	50–150
methadone/Dolophine	10–80
morphine sulfate+naltrexone HCl/ Embeda (ER)	20/.08–100/4.0
oxycodone/OxyContin	20–320
oxymorphone HCl/Opana (ER)	10+
pregabalin/Lyrica	150–300
propoxyphene/Darvon	195–390
sumatriptan/Imitrex (for migraines)	25–50
sumatriptan + naproxen/Treximet	85/500

ADHD Medications/CNS Stimulants

atomoxetine/Strattera	40–80
caffeine	—
cocaine	—
dexmethylphenidate/Focalin (ER)	5–20
dextroamphetamine/ Dexedrine	5–40
dextroamphetamine + amphetamine/Adderall	2.5–40
guanfacine/Intuniv (ER)	1–4
lisdexamfetamine dimesylate/Vyvanse (ER) (prodrug)	20–70
methamphetamine/Methedrine/Desoxyn	5–25
methylphenidate/Ritalin/Concerta	5–50
Daytrana (transdermal)	10–30
modafinil/Provigil	100–200
nicotine	—

Nootropic Medications

donepezil/Aricept	5–10
galantamine/Reminyl	16–24
memantine/Namenda	20
rivastigmine/Exelon	3–12

Bipolar Disorder Medications

asenapine/Saphris (sublingual)	10–20
lithium/Eskalith/Lithobid	600–2400
lamotrigine/Lamictal	100–400
N-acetyl cysteine (add-on for dresspive symptons)	2grams
olanzapine+fluoxetine/Symbyax	6/25–12/50
Protein kinase C inhibitors(under study for mania)	
risperidone/Risperdal	4–16
sumatriptan (under study for bipolar disorder)	

Many atypical antipsychotic drugs are approved for use in bipolar disorder, particularly to treat manic episodes.

Anticonvulsants for Mania

carbamazepine/Tegretol	600–1600
topiramate/Topamax	25–400
valproate/Depakene/Depakote	750

Antipsychotic Medications

First Generation Antipsychotics (FGAs)

chlorpromazine/Thorazine	50–1500
fluphenazine/Prolixin	3–45
haloperidol/Haldol	2–40
perphenazine/Trilafon	8–60

Second Generation Antipsychotics (SGAs)

amoxapine/Ascendin	200–300
asenapine/Saphris (sublingual)	10–20
clozapine/Clozaril	300–900
olanzapine/Zyprexa/	5–20
Zydiss (soluble on tongue)	6
paliperidone/Invega (ER)	25–400
quetiapine/Seroquel	4–16
risperidone/Risperdal/Consta (i.m.)	40–160
ziprasidone/Geodon	

Dopamine System Stabilizers (DSSs)

aripiprazole/Abilify	10–30

Antidepressant Medications

Selective Serotonin Reuptake Inhibitors (SSRIs)

citalopram/Celexa	10–60
desvenlafaxine/Pristiq (ER)	50
escitalopram/Lexapro	10
fluoxetine/Prozac/Sarafem	10–80
fluvoxamine/Luvox (also ER)	50–300
(for OCD & Social AD)	
paroxetine/Paxil/Pexeva	10–60
sertraline/Zoloft	25–200
venlafaxine/Effexor (also ER)	75–375
(an SNRI at higher doses)	

Tricyclic & Heterocyclic Antidepressants (TCAs & HCAs)

amitriptyline/Elavil	50–300
clomipramine/Anafranil	25–250
desipramine/Norpramin	100–300
doxepin/Sinequan/Adapin	100–300
imipramine/Tofranil	25–300
nortriptyline/Aventyl/Pamelor	50–150

Monoamine Oxidase Inhibitors (MAOIs)

phenelzine/Nardil	30–90
tranylcypromine/Parnate	20–60
selegiline/Emsam (transdermal)	5–20

Atypical Antidepressants

aprepitant/Emend (not yet available)	
aripiprazole/Abilify (adjunctive treatment)	
bupropion/Aplenzin (ER)	522
bupropion/Wellbutrin/Zyban	200–450
duloxetine/Cymbalta	60
mirtazapine/Remeron	15–45
trazodone/Desyrel	200–400

Other Treatments for Dementia

- acetylcysteine
- ampakines (may improve cognition)
- antiamyloid treatments (gene therapy or vaccines)
- antioxidants
- COX-2 inhibitors (anti-inflammatory agents)
- ginkgo (increases blood flow to CNS)
- hormone replacement therapy (estrogens or androgens)
- huperzine/HupA (ACh esterase inhibitor)
- L-methylfolate
- neurotropic agents (human nerve growth factor)
- nicotine (stimulates ACh)
- NSAIDs (nonsteroidal anti-inflammatory drugs)
- Omega-3 fish oils
- phosphotidylserine/PtdSer (natural fat-soluble nutrient)
- selegiline/Eldepryl (MAO inhibitor)
- statin drugs (lower cholesterol)
- vitamin B3 (niacin)
- vitamin C (antioxidant)
- vitamin E (antioxidant)

Miscellaneous Medications

acamprosate/Campral	1998
benztropine/Cogentin	150–250
disulfiram/Antabuse	125–500
naloxone/Narcan (i.v.)	.04–2
naltrexone/Trexan/Revia	25–150
nizatidine/Axid	75–300
ondansetron/Zofran	4–300
sildenafil/Viagra	25–100
varenicline/Chantix (anti smoking)	0.5–1.0
sodium oxybate/Xyrem	4.5–9 (grams)
(for narcolepsy)	

All doses are oral unless indicated.

THIS IS NOT A COMPLETE LIST.
See www.rxlist.com for up-to-date information on prescription drugs.

Drugs & Clients™

What Every Psychotherapist Needs to Know

Padma Catell, PhD

www.drugsandclients.com

Index

About the Author

Padma Catell, PhD, is Professor Emerita of Psychology at the California Institute of Integral Studies and a licensed Psychologist. She earned her BA in Biology at Hunter College and an MA in Biology at the City University of New York with a specialization in pharmacology, which she studied at the Mount Sinai School of Medicine. She has been teaching psychopharmacology at CIIS, Dominican University, and other graduate schools in the San Francisco Bay area since 1984. Her advanced

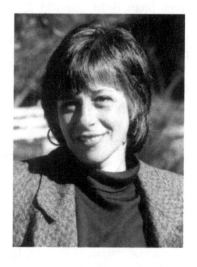

degrees in both biology and psychology, combined with extensive teaching and clinical experience, make Dr. Catell uniquely qualified to understand and address the problems facing today's psychotherapists and other health-care professionals in this rapidly-changing, highly-controversial, and increasingly-important area of psychology.

Psychopharmacology for Psychotherapists

Drugs and Clients: What Every Psychotherapist Needs to Know (2nd. edition)

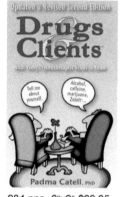

This textbook is for all psychotherapists, psychology students and instructors as well as all health-care professionals, including doctors, nurses, counselors, and social workers, who are not trained in the specialty of psychiatry — $39.95.

Attention Educators! For a detailed course outline illustrating how Dr. Catell uses the text in her psychopharmacology classes, visit the website and click on the "For Educators" link.

Reference Card   8.5" X 11" card — only $7.95

284 pps. 6"x9" $39.95
ISBN: 978-0929150-789

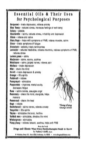 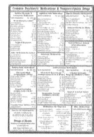

This handy reference card includes two tables from the book, Common Psychiatric Medications (pp. 256–257) and Psychological Uses of Essential Oils (p. 210), enlarged and printed in full color on sturdy 8.5" X 11" card stock.

Through the Gateway of the Heart (2nd. edition)

Accounts of Experiences with MDMA and other Empathogenic Substances.

Includes a new Preface by Padma Catell, Foreword by Ralph Metzner, and Revised Guidelines for the Sacramental Use of Empathogenic Substances.

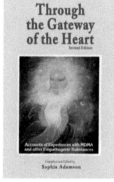

202 pps. 6"x9" $25.00
ISBN: 978-0929150-79-6
eBook $12.99

This book, which was originally published in 1985 before MDMA became illegal, is a compilation of over forty personal experiences with MDMA conducted in supportive and/or therapeutic settings. The vignettes illustrate MDMA's potential in generating insight, facilitating empathic communication, and supporting spiritual practice. Although the use of MDMA remains illegal (except in the limited context of approved research), the editors of this book, like many psychotherapy professionals, believe that a fresh look at this very promising substance is warranted.

Free Reference Card & Free Postage & Handling

Receive a free reference card and free P&H with any book purchased directly from Solarium Press. www.drugsandclients.com • 800-777-9977

CPSIA information can be obtained
at www.ICGtesting.com
Printed in the USA
FSHW020521290119
55323FS